A B C OF HYPERTENSION

A B C OF HYPERTENSION

Published by the British Medical Association
Tavistock Square, London WC1H 9JR

First Edition 1981
Fifth Impression 1985
Second Edition 1987
Second Impression 1988
Third Impression 1988
Fourth Impression 1988
Fifth Impression 1989
Sixth Impression 1990
Seventh Impression 1991

ISBN 0-7279-0193-1

PRINTED IN NORTHERN IRELAND AT THE UNIVERSITIES PRESS (BELFAST) LTD.
Typesetting by Latimer Trend & Company Ltd, Plymouth.

Contents

Page

The illustration on the back cover of Stephen Hales measuring the blood pressure in a horse is reproduced from the *Medical Times* of 1944.

Preface

It is five years since the first version of the *ABC of Hypertension* was published in series format in the *British Medical Journal*. Since that time a great deal of new information has become available, and many sections of the original series are now obsolete. The aim of the series was and still is to provide a safe main stream approach to hypertension, which is the most common chronic disease requiring treatment, and to avoid contentious issues. A framework for the management of hypertension both in general practice and hospitals is necessary; the results of recent clinical trials and the introduction of new drugs have meant that some rethinking of the approach has had to be done.

Sadly, many of the problems prevalent five years ago are still major issues. In particular, ample evidence indicates that in Britain and other Western countries hypertension is still underdiagnosed and undertreated. We can, however, be encouraged by the increasing number of reports of prospective case detection programmes based on primary health care teams. Although some hypertensive patients do require hospital referral, most can be managed exclusively in general practice. It is hoped that the updated *ABC* will help to improve the rate of detection and management of hypertension.

D G BEEVERS 1987
Reader in Medicine,
Dudley Road Hospital,
Birmingham

THE OBSERVER

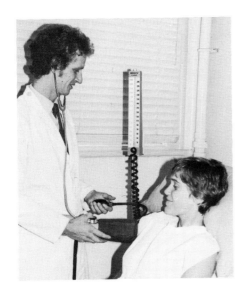

Apart from the stethoscope, the sphygmomanometer is probably used more than any other single instrument both in hospital and general practice. Doctors, nurses, and paramedical staff record blood pressure; and decisions on treatment, investigation, prognosis, fitness for insurance and employment, and epidemiological conclusions are based on these measurements. Patients themselves are often trained to record their own blood pressure, and machines which record blood pressure may be found in some shops and airports.

When blood pressure is measured by routine sphygmomanometry the reading is generally assumed to be accurate, and little thought is given to major errors that may arise through inadequate knowledge, carelessness, or poor maintenance of the instrument. Many doctors and nurses are unaware of potential errors of technique and fail to appreciate the limits of blood pressure measurement. They may therefore attach undue clinical importance to what is, at best, an inaccurate technique of measurement.

Training

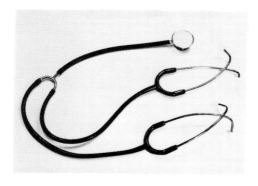

There is a surprising degree of variation in blood pressure interpretation among observers. Much of the variation is probably due to failure to appreciate that if indirect sphygmomanometry is to be accurate attention to detail, especially in interpreting sounds, is essential.

Nurses and medical students are often inadequately trained in blood pressure measurement. With increasing reliance on paramedical staff for recording blood pressure and the increasing interest in home recording of blood pressure much more attention needs to be directed towards training methods. Audiovisual techniques are ideally suited both to showing and to assessing blood pressure measurement, and are helpful for training students and nurses. These techniques are costly, however, and are not always readily available for training patients or their relatives. It is surprising how proficient patients (and students) may become in measuring blood pressure using illustrated written instructions. None the less, accuracy should not be taken for granted, and the trainee's ability to measure pressure accurately should be assessed carefully with a dual stethoscope.

What biases the observer?

History and risk factors

Age

Drug trial

Blood pressure trial

The observer is often unconsciously biased towards raising or lowering the patient's blood pressure. This is most likely to occur when there is an arbitrary division between normal and high blood pressure, such as 140/90 mm Hg. An observer might tend to record a favourable measurement in a young healthy man with a borderline increase in pressure but categorise as hypertensive an obese, middle aged man with a similar reading. Likewise, there might be observer bias in overreading blood pressure to include the patient in a study, such as a drug trial. Adequate discussion during training to make the observer aware of this sort of bias might minimise its influence.

The observer

Terminal digit preference

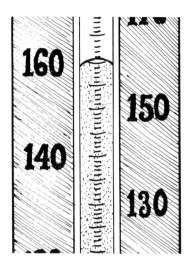

Observers show a strong preference for the terminal digits 0 and 5, even though a 5 mm marking does not appear on many scales. There is some evidence that careful training may minimise this source of error; and if the observer can devote enough time to recording the blood pressure and if the scale is clearly marked the pressure may be recorded to the nearest 2 mm Hg. The Hawksley random zero sphygmomanometer is used in research to reduce the effect of observer bias.

Viewing distance and angle

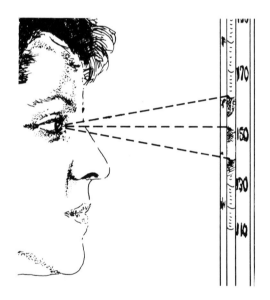

The observer should be no further than three feet from the manometer so that he can read the scale easily.

The mercury manometer has a vertical scale and errors will occur unless the eye is kept close to the level of the meniscus.

The aneroid scale is a composite of vertical and horizontal divisions and numbers and must be viewed straight on—with the eye on a line perpendicular to the centre of the face of the gauge.

Taking care and time

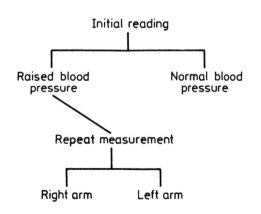

The observer should be in a comfortable relaxed position. If he is hurried he will release the pressure too rapidly and will thus underestimate the systolic pressure and overestimate the diastolic. If he is interrupted he may forget the exact measurement and estimate it, causing an inaccurate value to be recorded. The blood pressure reading should be written as soon as it is measured because relying on memory may result in error.

It takes about five minutes to measure blood pressure accurately, but in practice considerably less time is devoted to the procedure. If the blood pressure is raised at the initial assessment the observer should repeat the measurement and also take the blood pressure in the other arm.

Partial loss of hearing is another potential source of error. Low energy acoustic sounds, such as the Korotkov sounds, may be just above the normal hearing threshold when listened for with a stethoscope, and an observer may not recognise his inability to appreciate these sounds. Periodic assessment of staff with a dual stethoscope or audiovisual tests will detect hearing deficits and other alterations in the technique of measurement that may cause inaccuracy.

THE SPHYGMOMANOMETER

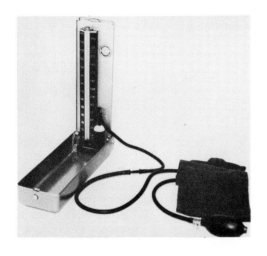

The sphygmomanometer is an indispensable piece of medical diagnostic equipment, but all too often its continuing efficiency is taken for granted. A survey of our hospital sphygmomanometers showed that nearly half of them were inaccurate, and similar results have been found in other hospitals. The proportion is similar in general practice. Few hospitals have any policy for the regular maintenance of basic equipment such as sphygmomanometers.

Mercury manometers

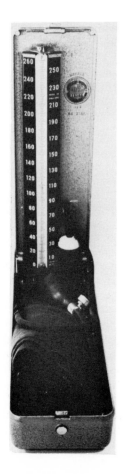

Mercury sphygmomanometers are reliable pieces of equipment that are easily maintained. Assessed against direct intra-arterial pressures, the standard mercury-in-glass manometer tends to underestimate slightly systolic pressure and overestimate diastolic (phase 5) pressure.

The top of the mercury meniscus should rest at exactly zero without pressure applied; if it is below this mercury needs to be added to the reservoir. The scale should be clearly calibrated in 2 mm divisions from 0 to 300 mm Hg (we hope kilopascals will not be introduced) and should indicate accurately the differences between the levels of mercury in the tube and in the reservoir. The diameter of the reservoir must be at least 10 times that of the vertical tube, or the vertical scale must correct for the drop in the mercury level in the reservoir as the column rises.

Substantial errors may occur if the manometer is not kept vertical during measurement. (Calibrations on floor models are especially adjusted to compensate for the tilt in the face of the gauge.)

The air vent at the top of the manometer must be kept patent as clogging will cause the mercury column to respond sluggishly to pressure changes. Mercury sphygmomanometers need cleaning and checking every six to 12 months, depending on use.

The mercury sphygmomanometer is the simplest and most accurate device for the indirect measurement of blood pressure and must be recommended for general clinical use. It can be maintained and serviced easily without having to be returned to the supplier.

The sphygmomanometer

Aneroid manometers

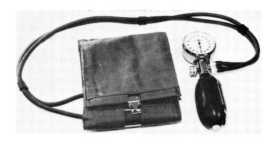

Aneroid sphygmomanometers have levers which can stick and are affected by jolts, and they are generally less accurate than mercury manometers. When calibrated against a mercury manometer an average deviation of 3 mm Hg is considered to be acceptable. Even so, some studies have shown that 30–35% of aneroid sphygmomanometers have an average deviation of over 3 mm Hg, while 6–13% deviate by 7 mm Hg or more.

Some new aneroid sphygmomanometers incorporate a gauge which indicates when the machine is losing accuracy.

Aneroid manometers need to be checked every six months against an accurate mercury manometer over the entire pressure range. If inaccuracies or other faults are found the instrument must be returned to the manufacturers or supplier for repair.

Which manometer?

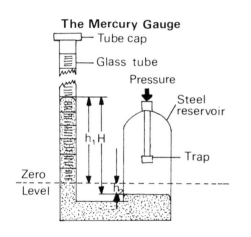

The Mercury Gauge

- Tube cap
- Glass tube
- Pressure
- Steel reservoir
- Trap
- Zero Level
- $h_1 H$
- h_2

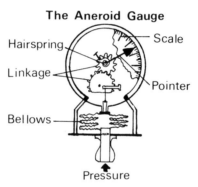

The Aneroid Gauge

- Hairspring
- Linkage
- Bellows
- Scale
- Pointer
- Pressure

Adapted from illustrations in *The Baumonometer Service Manual*. New York: WA Baum & Co.

The choice of sphygmomanometer should be influenced by the use to which it will be put, the care with which it will be treated, and the availability of facilities for regular maintenance. When a machine will be used by many observers and is therefore likely to be knocked or jolted, and when maintenance facilities are not available, the mercury sphygmomanometer is better than the aneroid machine.

For the measurement of blood pressures in hospital wards a mercury sphygmomanometer on a stand with wheels is recommended. This allows the observer to adjust the level of the sphygmomanometer and to perform the measurement without having to balance the sphygmomanometer precariously on the side of the bed.

The cuff

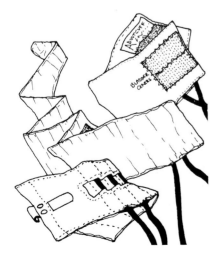

The cuff is an inelastic cloth that encircles the arm and encloses the inflatable rubber bladder. It is secured round the arm most commonly by Velcro tape, occasionally by wrapping a tapering end into the encircling cuff, and rarely by hooks.

Tapering cuffs should be long enough to encircle the arm several times: the full length should extend beyond the end of the inflatable bladder for 25 cm and then should gradually taper for a further 60 cm. Velcro surfaces must be effective, and when they lose their grip the cuff should be discarded.

The inflatable bladder

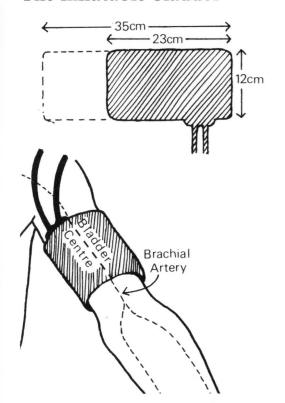

A bladder which is too short or too narrow, or both (overall too small), will give falsely high pressures, and one which is too wide or too long, or both (overall too large), will give falsely low pressures. Nevertheless, if the bladder is too wide or too narrow inaccuracy will be reduced provided that the bladder is long enough to encircle the arm completely. Readings taken with a completely encircling bladder correlate best with intra-arterial pressure.

The recommended bladder width is 20% greater than (or 1·2 times) the diameter of the limb, which is equivalent to 40% of the arm's circumference. Most bladders are 12 to 13 cm wide, with those for obese arms being 15 or 16 cm, but most arms will not comfortably accommodate a cuff much wider than 13 cm.

Bladder lengths vary from around 22 to 36 cm, there being different lengths for obese arms, for children's arms, and for thighs. The standard bladder (22·9 cm long) will encircle only 33% of adult arms, whereas a 36 cm bladder would encircle 99% of adult arms.

Manufacturers of blood pressure equipment must be persuaded to review bladder size. We recommend that for adults the bladder should be 35 cm long and 12 cm wide.

If the bladder does not encircle the arm, the centre of the bladder must be placed directly over the artery to be compressed, or the readings will be very inaccurate. Many cuffs now indicate the centre of the bladder and also indicate bladder size in relation to arm circumference.

Rubber tubing, pump, and control valve

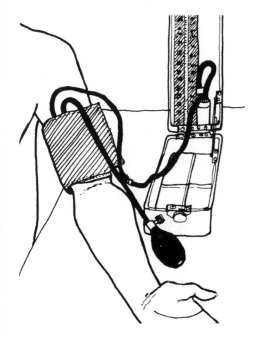

Leaks due to cracked or perished rubber make accurate measurement of the blood pressure difficult because the fall in mercury cannot be controlled. The rubber should be in a good condition and free of leaks. The tubing should be at least 76 cm long, and connections must be airtight and easily disconnected.

The control valve is a common source of error, especially in sphygmomanometers with an air filter, rather than a rubber valve. The filter may become blocked with dirt, which demands excessive squeeze on the pump. The control valve should allow the passage of air without excessive effort; when closed it should hold the mercury at a constant level; and when released it should allow a controlled fall in the level of mercury.

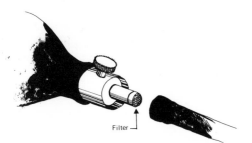

The valve may be tested by rolling a cloth cuff into its own tail or, with a Velcro cuff, matching Velcro to Velcro, and then pumping up to 200 mm Hg and waiting for 10 seconds. The mercury should not fall more than 2 mm Hg during those 10 seconds. If it does fall further the circuit should be clamped in sections to locate the leak, which is usually in the control valve. The valve should then be released slowly four times, on two of which it should be possible to control the rate of fall to 1 mm Hg per second, and to change from faster to slower rates at will. Inability to do so is usually due to air filter blockage, which may be rectified by cleaning the filter, but in practice it is usually simpler to replace the pump and control valve.

The sphygmomanometer

The Hawksley random zero sphygmomanometer

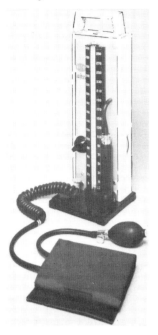

Blood pressure measurement with a standard mercury sphygmomanometer is inadequate for research work because observer bias is easily introduced. To minimise this the Hawksley random zero sphygmomanometer is used in research studies. This device is only slightly larger than the conventional sphygmomanometer and operates in the same way, except that a wheel is spun before each measurement to adjust the zero to an unknown level. Once the blood pressure has been measured the level of zero may be determined and the pressure reading corrected.

In this way observer bias is reduced but not digit preference. The machine compares favourably with the standard mercury manometer and direct intra-arterial pressure.

Maintenance

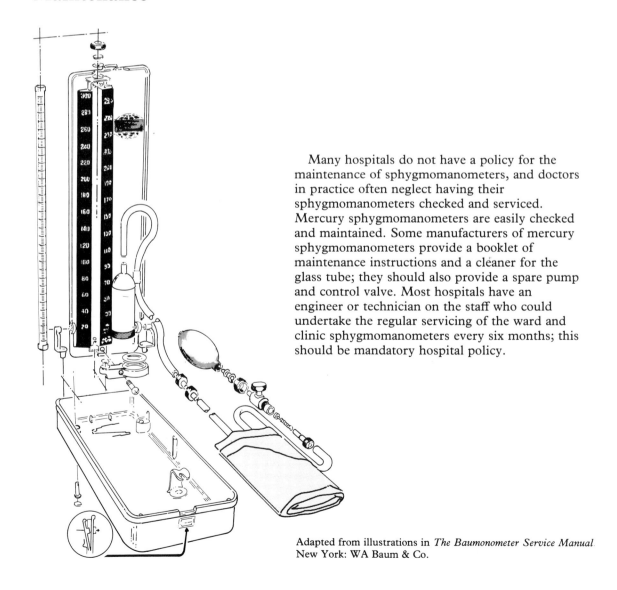

Many hospitals do not have a policy for the maintenance of sphygmomanometers, and doctors in practice often neglect having their sphygmomanometers checked and serviced. Mercury sphygmomanometers are easily checked and maintained. Some manufacturers of mercury sphygmomanometers provide a booklet of maintenance instructions and a cleaner for the glass tube; they should also provide a spare pump and control valve. Most hospitals have an engineer or technician on the staff who could undertake the regular servicing of the ward and clinic sphygmomanometers every six months; this should be mandatory hospital policy.

Adapted from illustrations in *The Baumonometer Service Manual* New York: WA Baum & Co.

Semiautomated sphygmomanometers

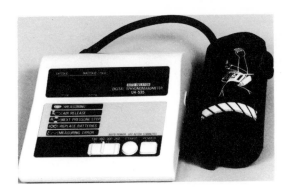

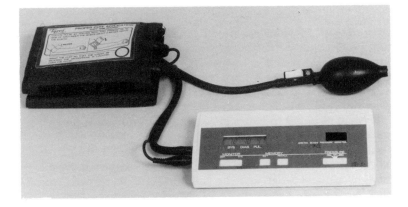

The auscultatory method of measuring blood pressure is accurate enough for clinical practice if the observer is adequately trained and minimises error by attention to detail. Several semiautomated devices are available on the market that claim to be more accurate than conventional mercury or aneroid sphygmomanometers.

The basic assumption made by many manufacturers of these machines (and by some of the public and medical staff who use them) is that automation will improve the accuracy of measurement. Nevertheless, many of these machines, which are much more expensive than a standard mercury manometer, are not as accurate. Most semiautomated devices incorporate some form of audiovisual signalling of end points, and some possess automatic control of inflation or deflation, or both. Some also provide a permanent record of the blood pressure, a facility which may reduce observer bias and error. Nevertheless, technical details on these machines are often lacking and the end point selected for diastolic pressure may not be clearly defined.

Most semiautomated machines work on one of two principles—the detection of Korotkov sounds (by human ear or a microphone) or the detection of arterial blood flow by ultrasound.

Photographs of the semiautomated sphygmomanometers are reproduced by kind permission of the Royal College of Surgeons.

A number of semiautomated devices based on Korotkov sound detection are available. An electronic microphone shielded from extraneous noise in the pressure cuff will detect the Korotkov sounds and indicate the pressure on a chart, or audiovisually by bleeps or blinking lights. The microphones are sensitive to movement and friction, however, and are difficult to place accurately. Manual or automatic inflation and deflation, or both, may be available.

Other techniques being developed include the phase-shift method, which measures pressure changes between two segments of a double cuff; infrasound recording; oscillographic detection of arterial pulsations with a double arm cuff; tonometry, which depends on the principle that displacement of a force sensitive transducer over a superficial artery can be made linearly proportional to the arterial blood pressure.

Complex devices that record blood pressure automatically at preset intervals have been designed for intensive care units and theatres. These devices often use two methods of measurement, most commonly Korotkov sound detection and oscillometry, but often the mode being used is not indicated and assessments of accuracy for each mode are sometimes not available from the manufacturers. Moreover, these units do not always lend themselves to independent assessments of accuracy because of their complex design. Reports of accuracy, often inconclusive or conflicting, appear sporadically in the public reports from independent research units, but it may be many years before there is sufficient evidence to enable prospective buyers to make a confident judgment. Directors of intensive care units and anaesthetists buying theatre equipment should seek stringent documentation of accuracy from manufacturers before buying these devices, which may be priced from £2000 to £5000.

THE PATIENT

A person's blood pressure varies from moment to moment with respiration, emotion, exercise, meals, tobacco, alcohol, temperature, bladder distension, and pain, and it is influenced by changes in circadian rhythms, age, and race. Furthermore, the patient may have physical characteristics such as obesity, or diseases which may modify the blood pressure or make its measurement difficult or inaccurate. We cannot standardise our patients but we can minimise the effect of environmental influences by taking account of such factors.

Anxiety raises blood pressure, often by as much as 30 mm Hg, and the doctor may prove a potent cause of raised blood pressure, a phenomenon aptly described as "white coat hypertension." Adequate explanation of the procedure is important to allay the fears of anxious patients. It is essential if the patient with hypertension is to take part in the management of his or her disease and adhere to treatment. Home recording of blood pressure is becoming an important part of management.

Patients should avoid exertion and not eat or smoke for 30 minutes before having their blood pressure measured. The room should be comfortably warm and quiet, and the patient should be allowed to rest for at least five minutes before the measurement. When it is not possible to achieve optimum conditions this should be noted with the blood pressure reading—for example, "BP 150/95/90 R arm, V phase (patient very nervous)."

Age	Alcohol
Race	Smoking
Temperature	Exercise
Pain	Illness
Emotion	Obesity

Obesity

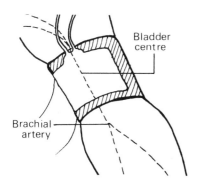

Bladder centre

Brachial artery

High blood pressure is commoner in obese people, but this increase may be at least partly artefactual, as the inflatable rubber bladder may be too short for the obese arm—causing "cuff hypertension." Ideally the bladder should encircle the arm, the recommended dimensions being 12 × 35 cm, but if the bladder does not do so (and most do not) it should be 1·2 times wider than the arm's diameter (or 40% of arm circumference). When the bladder does not completely encircle the arm the centre of the bladder must be placed directly over the brachial artery.

Arrhythmias

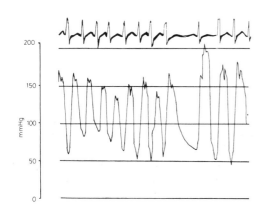

Many cardiac arrhythmias cause variations in stroke volume, and the blood pressure may vary with each cardiac contraction. This is particularly so with atrial fibrillation. The average of at least three readings should be recorded for both systolic and diastolic pressure, and a note of the arrhythmia should be made with the blood pressure reading. The mercury should be lowered very slowly to avoid underestimating systolic and overestimating diastolic pressures.

Arm position and support

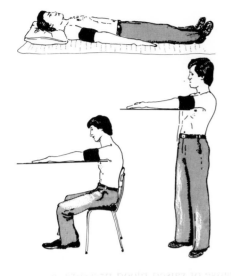

In normal people there is no major difference in blood pressure between supine, sitting, and standing positions provided that the arm is supported at heart level. Patients should be comfortable whatever their position, and they should not change their position for five minutes before the blood pressure is measured. Some antihypertensive drugs cause postural hypertension, and when this is expected blood pressure should be measured both lying and standing.

Vertical displacement of the arm increases the hydrostatic pressure as the arm is lowered. The error may be as large as 10 mm Hg for both the systolic and diastolic pressures. The arm in which pressure is being measured should be horizontal with the fourth intercostal space at the sternum. This is especially important in the sitting and standing positions: in the supine position the arm is usually at heart level.

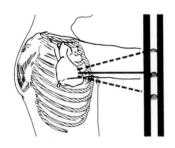

If the arm is unsupported the patient will perform isometric exercise, which may increase diastolic pressure by up to 10%. This effect is greater in hypertensive patients and in those taking β adrenoceptor blocking drugs. This isometric effect is most likely to occur in sitting and standing positions, when the arm has been extended forward at an angle of 45° to keep it at heart level. When extended this way the arm can readily be supported by the observer's arm.

Which arm?

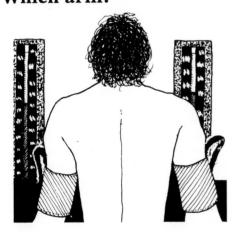

There may be differences in pressure between arms, but in practice these are rarely important. In clinical practice most pressures are recorded from the right side.

At the initial examination, however, the blood pressure should be estimated in both arms. If there are differences greater than 20 mm Hg for systolic or 10 mm Hg for diastolic pressure on three consecutive readings simultaneous measurement should be carried out to determine if the difference is real or artefactual. This is done by two trained observers recording the blood pressure simultaneously in both arms using one sphygmomanometer connected by a Y connector to two occluding cuffs.

Repeated measurements

1 Inflate rapidly to 30 mm Hg above systolic
2 Deflate at 2 mm Hg / second
3 Note: appearance of sounds (systolic)
      muffling of sounds
      disappearance of sounds (diastolic)
4 Deflate rapidly to zero
5 Wait ≥ 15 seconds before repeating measurement

Repeated inflation of the bladder causes venous congestion of the limb, the duration of inflation rather than the pressure being the important factor. Systolic pressure may be up to 30 mm Hg above or 14 mm Hg below the true arterial level, and diastolic readings may be up to 20 mm Hg above or 10 mm Hg below the true level. To avoid venous congestion the cuff should be inflated as rapidly as possible and then deflated completely between successive readings. At least 15 seconds should be allowed between successive measurements.

TECHNIQUE

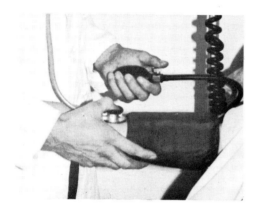

Indirect blood pressure measurement by auscultation is susceptible to several errors, which may originate with the observer, the sphygmomanometer, the patient, or a combination of these factors.

By careful attention to detail blood pressure measurement with a sphygmomanometer can give systolic and diastolic pressures within 4 mm Hg of intra-arterial pressures.

Korotkov sounds

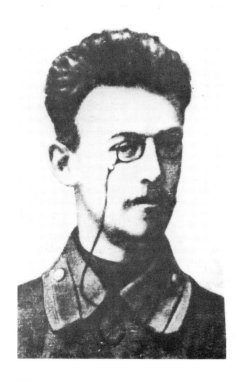

Shortly after Scipione Riva-Rocci had invented the sphygmomanometer a Russian surgeon, Dr N C Korotkov (left), reported that by placing a stethoscope over the brachial artery at the antecubital fossa distal to the Riva-Rocci cuff, sounds could be heard. He documented the phases, and thus introduced the indirect ausculatory method of recording blood pressure.

Although the origin of the Korotkov sounds is still not clear, vibratory and flow phenomena are probably responsible.

The phases are:

Phase 1—The first appearance of faint clear tapping sounds which gradually increase in intensity. The systolic pressure is heard for at least two consecutive beats, and this correlates well with intra-arterial pressure.

Phase 2—The softening of sounds, which may become swishing.

Phase 3—The return of sharper sounds, which become crisper but never fully regain the intensity of phase 1 sounds. Neither phase 2 nor phase 3 has any known clinical importance.

Phase 4—The distinct abrupt muffling of sounds, which become soft and blowing.

Phase 5—The point at which all sounds disappear completely.

Diastolic dilemma

Recommendations		Phase
1939	Cardiac Society of Great Britain and Ireland and American Heart Association (AHA)	4
1951	AHA	5
1959	Build and Blood Pressure Study	5
1962	WHO	4 & 5
1967	AHA	4
1970	Veterans Administration Study	5
1972	Hypertension Detection and Follow up Study	5
1974	Framingham Study	4
1975	Medical Research Council	5
1981	AHA	5
1985	British Hypertension Society	5

Recommendations on blood pressure measurement have vacilated for many years on the issue of the diastolic end point. In the United States of America doctors have tended to favour the silent end point (phase 5), whereas in Britain and Ireland they have favoured the muffled end point (phase 4). In 1962 the World Health Organisation recommended that both phases 4 and 5 should be recorded. Inability to decide on an empirical matter of such importance is a source of inaccuracy and confusion.

Muffling and the disappearance of sounds may be synchronous, but usually there is a difference of 5 to 10 mm Hg. Phase 5 correlates best with intra-arterial pressure, but general acceptance of the silent end point has been resisted because patients in whom flow within the arterial circulation is increased—for example, after exercise and in other high output states—may have a silent end point greatly below the muffling of sounds. In some patients sounds may be audible when cuff pressure is deflated even to zero. On the other hand, some patients do not have a distinct muffled end point.

There is greater agreement between observers using the silent rather than the muffled end point—a matter of importance in training observers, be they patients, nurses, or doctors. We recommend that the silent end point (phase 5) should be taken as the diastolic pressure, except in pregnancy when the muffled (phase 4) end point is taken, because in many pregnant women the silent end point is greatly below muffling of the sounds. To avoid confusion, however, we support the suggestion that the fourth and fifth phases should always be noted—for example, 160/95/65 mm Hg, or when only the fourth or fifth phase has been recorded 160/95/- mm Hg or 160/-/65 mm Hg, respectively.

Technique

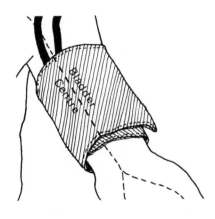

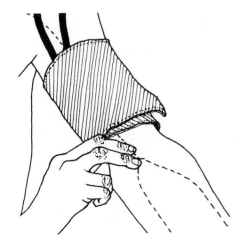

Firstly, the factors already discussed in relation to the observer, the instrument, and the patient should be taken into account.

Secondly, all clothing should be removed from the arm. If a blouse, shirt, or pyjama jacket is not to be removed it is better to leave the cloth under the cuff than roll the sleeve into a constricting band. If the cuff is not applied snugly to the arm falsely high blood pressures will be recorded, and if the cuff is too tight errors will also occur.

Thirdly, the cuff should be wrapped round the arm ensuring that the bladder dimensions are accurate. If the bladder does not completely encircle the arm the centre of the bladder must be over the brachial artery. The rubber tubes from the bladder are usually placed inferiorly, often at the site of the brachial artery, but we suggest that they should be placed superiorly or, with completely encircling bladders, posteriorly, so that the antecubital fossa is easily accessible for auscultation.

Fourthly, the brachial artery should be palpated with one hand, and the cuff rapidly inflated to about 30 mm Hg above the disappearance of the pulse and then slowly deflated. The observer should note the pressure at which the pulse reappears. This is the approximate level of the systolic pressure, and because phase 1 sounds sometimes disappear as pressure is reduced and reappear at a lower level (the auscultatory gap), the systolic pressure may be underestimated unless already determined by palpation. (The radial artery is often used for palpatory estimation of the systolic pressure but by using the brachial artery the observer also establishes its location before auscultation.)

Technique

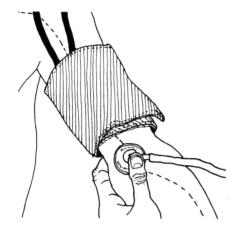

Fifthly, the stethoscope should be placed over the brachial artery. A bell end piece gives better sound reproduction, but a diaphragm is easier to secure with the fingers of one hand and covers a larger area. The stethoscope should be held firmly and evenly but without excessive pressure. Too much pressure may distort the artery, producing sounds below diastolic pressure. To avoid friction sounds the stethoscope end piece should not touch the clothing, cuff, or rubber tubes.

Sixthly, the cuff should be inflated rapidly to about 30 mm Hg above the palpated systolic pressure and deflated at a rate of 2 to 3 mm Hg per heart beat (or per second).

Seventhly, the appearance of sounds (phase 1) should be recorded as the systolic pressure, and the disappearance of sounds (phase 5) as the diastolic. Ideally both phases should be recorded, but this is especially important if the difference between phases is over 10 mm Hg.

Finally, pressures should be recorded to the nearest 2 mm Hg. When all sounds have disappeared the cuff should be deflated rapidly and completely before repeating the measurement to prevent venous congestion of the arm.

Repeated measurements

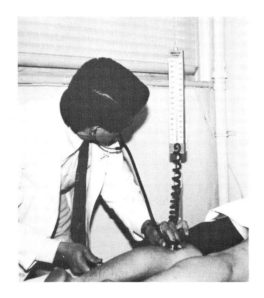

If the blood pressure is raised on first measurement the recording should be repeated. At an initial examination blood pressure should be measured in both arms. If the difference between arms is more than 20 mm Hg for systolic or 10 mm Hg for diastolic pressure simultaneous blood pressure measurement in both arms should be performed as described above.

Except when the initial measurement is very high, indicating urgent treatment, the blood pressure should be measured on at least two separate occasions before starting treatment or diagnosing "hypertension" because as many as half the patients with raised blood pressures on initial examination will become normotensive on subsequent examination, and both systolic and diastolic pressures will be overestimated if based on a single casual estimation rather than repeated examination. In practice many measurements of blood pressure are usually taken over many weeks or months before diagnostic and therapeutic decisions are made.

In patients with suspected coarctation of the aorta the blood pressure should be measured in the leg. A thigh cuff containing a large bladder (18 × 40 cm for adults) should be wrapped round the thigh of the prone patient and the Korotkov sounds auscultated in the popliteal fossa in the usual way. The pressure in the legs is normally equal to that in the arms if the bladder is adequate in size.

Ideally, therefore, records of blood pressure measurement should show the systolic pressure, the diastolic pressure, the end point used, the limb used and whether right or left, the position of the patient, and the presence of any arrhythmias or unusual circumstances such as anxiety or confinement to bed.

The photograph of Korotkov is reproduced by kind permission of Dr H Segall.

INFANCY AND CHILDHOOD

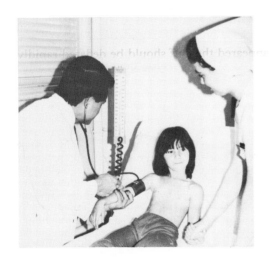

As in the adult, blood pressure measurement in children should be an indispensable part of clinical assessment, as doctors are becoming increasingly aware that hypertension may occur in childhood. If blood pressure readings in children are to be of value, however, the examiner must devote considerable care and time to the technique of measurement.

The physical stimuli affecting blood pressure—anxiety, fear, apprehension, agitation, activity, respiration, and temperature—are likely to be greater in children than in adults. The child must be relaxed, and in small children the observer may also have to allow for the effects of crying and restraint.

It is important in children to measure the blood pressure in the arms and legs. The systolic pressure in the leg is often said to be higher than in the arm, diastolic pressure being about the same, but any differences are probably due to inadequate cuff size.

Five main methods of measuring blood pressure in children have been used—auscultation, the flush method, visual oscillometry, palpation, and ultrasound. Impedance plethysmography has also been used, but clinical experience with the technique is limited. The auscultatory method is the commonest in children aged over 5 years, but in younger children and infants the Korotkov sounds are softer so that accurate interpretation becomes difficult and other techniques are necessary.

Auscultation

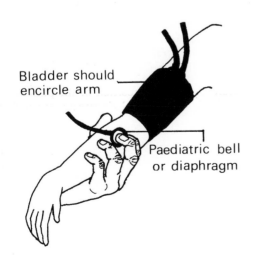

Bladder should encircle arm

Paediatric bell or diaphragm

The general recommendations on blood pressure measurement in the adult also apply to the child but a few points need emphasis.

Bladder size—Because of the variation in the size of the arm in children, choosing a cuff containing the correct bladder size is important. A bladder that is too narrow or too short will give an erroneously high pressure. One that is too wide or too long will have the opposite effect. An index for making a choice of the proper cuff is available but is rarely used. The bladder width should cover about two thirds of the length of the upper arm, and it should be long enough to encircle the arm completely. The length of the bladder is more important than width and if the optimal cuff is not available it is better to err with too large rather than too small a bladder. Paediatric units should have a selection of cuffs available. In hospital paediatric practice, where different observers may make serial observations, it is important to indicate bladder size with the blood pressure recording.

Stethoscope—The stethoscope used for auscultation should have a paediatric bell or diaphragm.

Diastolic end point—As with the adult, there is controversy whether muffling (phase 4) or disappearance (phase 5) of the Korotkov sounds is the better index of diastolic pressure. As the fifth phase may not occur at all in children, however, the muffled rather than the silent end point is generally recommended.

Palpation and visual oscillometry

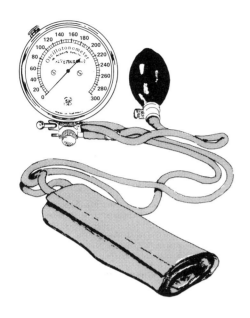

In the absence of ultrasound devices palpation of the arterial pressure distal to an occluding cuff may be the only means available for obtaining an estimate of blood pressure in small children and infants. The systolic pressure is the point of appearance of the pulse as the pressure in the bladder is reduced. The blood pressure measured by palpation is usually 5–10 mm Hg lower than that measured by auscultation.

Visual oscillometry was popular at the turn of the century but is not much practised now. Sensitive electronic oscillometers, however, are now being developed and may become important in clinical practice. The points at which oscillation appears and abruptly decreases as cuff pressure is lowered are taken as the systolic and diastolic pressures, respectively.

The flush method was once the standard clinical method of measuring blood pressure in the newborn and small infants. It has now been replaced by ultrasound techniques and is only of historic interest. The technique was based on the principle that if an extremity was drained of blood by compression it blanched and the mean arterial pressure could be detected by observing the pressure at which the extremity flushed.

Blood pressure measurement by ultrasound

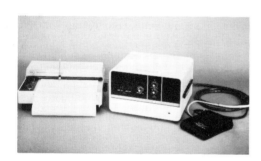

In small children and infants, in whom the Korotkov sounds may be soft, methods of measuring blood pressure that depend on hearing the sounds are not satisfactory. The same difficulty occurs in adults with low output states such as shock. Ultrasonic sphygmomanometry overcomes this problem and is now the method of choice for measuring blood pressure in small infants and the newborn.

The technique is based on the principle that an ultrasound wave directed towards an immobile structure such as an occluded artery will be reflected back without any change in frequency; a moving structure, such as the wall of a pulsating artery, will change the reflected wave and will vary with the velocity of blood flow.

A small transmitting and receiving ultrasound transducer is incorporated in an inflatable cuff, which is wrapped round the arm in the conventional manner so that the transducer overlies the brachial artery. When the cuff is inflated above systolic pressure the artery is occluded and the transmitted ultrasound waves are reflected back without any change in frequency. As the cuff is deflated the vessel opens and closes, producing frequency changes in the reflected ultrasound waves until the movement of the arterial wall ceases at the diastolic pressure, when the reflected ultrasound will again have a constant frequency. The variations in frequency of reflected ultrasound may be amplified to produce a signal that can be detected by headphones or speakers and recorded or displayed.

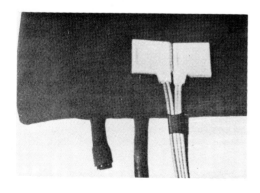

Although ultrasound is not influenced by environmental noise, the transmitting and receiving crystals must be accurately fixed and stable over the brachial artery. Even minor shifts in position will produce considerable inaccuracies. Ultrasound sphygmomanometers have proved reasonably reliable and accurate when assessed against standard sphygmomanometers and direct intra-arterial measurements, but the method is generally regarded as less accurate for diastolic than systolic pressure. The high cost of these instruments restricts their use.

The photograph of the Arteriosonde ultrasound machine was reproduced by kind permission of Kontron Medical and Laboratory Systems, St Albans.

FUTURE TRENDS

Blood pressure behaviour

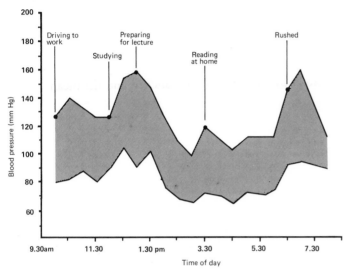

Variations in blood pressure with daily activity

Adapted from: Werdeyer D, Sokolow M, Parloff DB. *Trans Assoc Life Ins Med Dir Am* 1967; **51**: 93.

Previously decisions on the diagnosis, management, and prognosis of hypertension have been based for the greater part on occasional measurements of blood pressure, and in research conclusions on the efficacy of drugs have relied heavily on occasional measurements, usually taken at a particular time of the day. Techniques for measuring ambulatory blood pressure have shown that the variability of blood pressure, and decisions on the diagnosis, management, and prognosis of hypertension rely more on the pattern of blood pressure behaviour for a particular subject than on sporadic measurements of blood pressure. Likewise, an assessment of blood pressure behaviour is now generally incorporated into studies for assessing drugs that lower blood pressure.

Doctor recorded versus patient recorded measurement

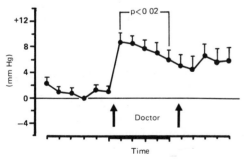

The rise in mean arterial pressure caused by a doctor's presence

Adapted from: Manuia G, Bertrini G, Grassi G, *et al. Clin Sci* 1982; **63**: 388.

It may be helpful in practice, and ultimately in understanding the behaviour of blood pressure, to break with the tradition of basing diagnostic and therapeutic decisions on a few isolated measurements of blood pressure. Blood pressure measurements may be taken under two sets of circumstances. Firstly, measurements made in the surgery, office, hospital clinic, or laboratory may be denoted as doctor recorded measurement; secondly, more active participation by the patient may be elicited in self recording and ambulatory measurement. With this classification, measurements recorded by patients are generally lower than those made by doctors. The consequence of this discrepancy in practice is that many people classified as hypertensive by the doctor's measurement will be normotensive by the patient's measurement.

Furthermore, doctor recorded measurements may fail to detect hypertensive patients at risk from cardiovascular complications. In conclusion, therefore, the time honoured method of measuring the blood pressure in the surgery or clinic may be less than ideal in the diagnosis, management, and prognosis of hypertension and should be supplemented by measurements recorded by the patient, be it a home recording or ambulatory measurement, or both.

Future trends

Methods for assessing blood pressure behaviour

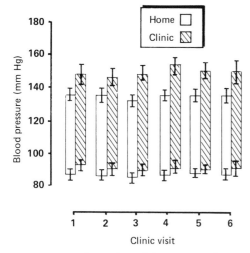

Comparison of the mean systolic and diastolic blood pressure in 21 patients measured at home and at hospital clinic at weekly intervals

Blood pressure behaviour may be assessed in three ways: firstly, and most simply, the blood pressure may be measured repeatedly and the pressures entered in a booklet or plotted against time; secondly, blood pressures may be recorded at home or at work by the patient, a friend, or relative; and, finally, the most comprehensive assessment of blood pressure behaviour may be obtained by ambulatory blood pressure measuring techniques.

Adapted from: *Baumonometer Service Manual.*
New York: WA Baum & Co. Inc.

Repeated blood pressure measurements

DATE	PLACE OF BP REC	TIME	BP S° D°	TABLETS NAME & STRENGTH	NUMBER AM	NUMBER PM
12/1/85	Hosp.	9.30 a.m.	144/94	Pressurex	5mg	—
16/1/85	Surgery	11am	168/104	Pressurex	5mg	—
24/1/85	Surgery	10.30am	144/106	Pressurex	5	5
1/2/85	Surgery	10.30a.	154/90	Pressurex	5	5
14/1/85	Hosp	10am	158/94	Pressurex / Diurex	5 / ⊤	5
20/1/85	Surgery	10.45	138/80	Pressurex / Diurex	5 / ⊤	5

Even with severe increases in blood pressure, decisions on treatment are seldom made on the basis of one or two blood pressure measurements, if for no other reason than to allow for the fall in blood pressure that occurs between visits. With mild and moderate hypertension there is no urgency to make a diagnosis of hypertension or initiate drug treatment. It is best to take several readings over a period of weeks, or even months, to obtain a pattern of blood pressure behaviour on which decisions can be firmly based and the effects of intervention subsequently judged. When indicated, blood pressure measurements can be obtained by trained staff using a standard mercury sphygmomanometer or semiautomated devices of confirmed accuracy over 12 or 16 hours in hospital; the readings, when plotted, give an assessment of daily blood pressure behaviour.

It is useful to provide hypertensive patients with a booklet, in which blood pressure measurements from all sources and changes of treatment may be entered. After a time this diary of blood pressure measurements becomes a valuable record of blood pressure behaviour.

Self measurement of blood pressure

Disadvantages:

- Patient unwilling to participate
- Patient unable to master technique
- Time required to train patient
- Time required to assess patient's accuracy
- Effects of observer bias and inaccuracy

Self measurement of blood pressure is a simple and economic means of obtaining a profile of blood pressure behaviour. Two disadvantages with the technique are that the patient may not wish to participate or may be unable to master the technique. Other disadvantages include the time needed to train and assess the patients' accuracy and the effect of observer bias and inaccuracy. In practice most patients may master the technique and achieve good accuracy from simple written and illustrated instructions. The doctor or other trained staff can test the subject's accuracy simply and quickly by connecting the two stethoscopes with a Y connector and checking the interpretation of the Korotkov sounds.

Name ██████████						
Drugs	PRESSUREX DIUREX					
Date	Blood pressure				Dose	
	am		pm			
	S	D	S	D	am	pm
1.9.79	174	104	210	112	80 2.5	80
2.9.79	200	108	212	110	80 2.5	80
3.9.79	198	104	222	116	80 2.5	80
4.9.79	202	100	206	105	80 2.5	80
5.9.79	186	98	198	100	80 2.5	80
6.9.79	176	94	180	98	80 2.5	80
7.9.79	180	90	180	94	80 2.5	80
8.9.79	190	98	204	104	100 2.5	100
9.9.79	164	92	190	106	100 2.5	100

Patients should record their own measurements of blood pressure in a booklet in the same way that the diabetic patient records the amount of sugar in the urine. In routine clinical practice a twice daily measurement of blood pressure twice a week will give a reasonable indication to both the patient and doctor of blood pressure control. When indicated, patients may record their blood pressure hourly or even half hourly over 12 hours to give a profile of daily blood pressure that correlates reasonably well with ambulatory blood pressure measurement.

The most accurate device for self measurement is the standard mercury sphygmomanometer with a cuff designed for easy application to the arm with one hand and which incorporates within the cloth a diaphragm stethoscope head. Aneroid devices are popular for self measurement of blood pressure, and the market boasts a large selection of semiautomated devices that are often expensive, and few of which have been tested for accuracy by an independent reputable laboratory. The main advantage of a semiautomated device with a microphone is that it removes the need for patient auscultation and should remove observer bias. Until manufacturers supply adequate information on accuracy for these devices, however, they cannot be recommended.

Ambulatory blood pressure measurement

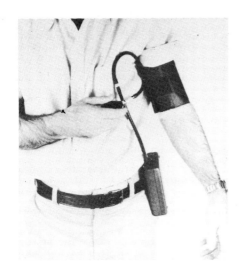

Ambulatory blood pressure may be measured continuously by direct intra-arterial techniques or intermittently with cuff occluding devices that are non-invasive. The complications, both potential and reported, with invasive direct recording of ambulatory blood pressure are formidable, and the technique must not be used in routine clinical practice. Several non-invasive systems giving intermittent blood pressure measurements over 12 to 24 hours are available, but all are extremely expensive and, as with all automated devices, a reputable assessment of accuracy is often not provided by the manufacturers. Consequently, independent researchers have to validate the equipment. The devices available record Korotkov sounds from a microphone positioned over the brachial artery below an occluding cuff, which may be inflated manually or automatically. Devices with automatic inflation have the advantage of being able to provide blood pressure measurements for 24 hours (usually taken every 30 minutes), whereas those with manual inflation provide recordings only during the waking hours, but these recorders are much lighter and preferred by patients.

Best results obtained by:

- Careful instructions to the patients

- Careful application of the equipment

- Regular maintenance of the equipment

- Careful decoding and presentation of the results

To obtain optimal results from the systems available considerable attention must be paid to instructions to the patient, application of the equipment, maintenance of the equipment, and decoding and presentation of results. This is best achieved by having a technician trained in ambulatory measurement, which adds considerably to the already high cost of this technique. Analysis of the data from ambulatory blood pressure measurement gives several calculations of blood pressure variability, which is helpful in determining the blood pressure load on the cardiovascular system and ultimately the prognosis for different forms of hypertension.

Future trends

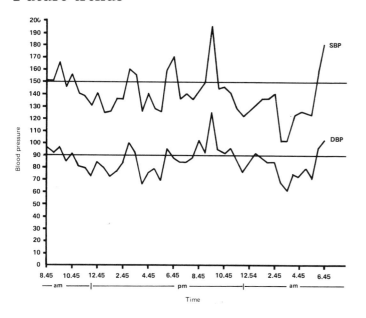

The plot of ambulatory blood pressure measurements against time gives a valuable "at a glance" assessment of blood pressure that helps in making decisions in borderline hypertension and in assessing the efficacy of antihypertensive drug treatment. The response of a patient's blood pressure to everyday stresses and activity may be examined by means of a diary card that is completed by the patient. Plots of ambulatory measurement serve to emphasise that casual blood pressure measurement, representing only about 1/1400 of the total day's blood pressure, may not only be unrepresentative but frankly misleading, particularly in patients with borderline or labile hypertension.

Based on a plot of ambulatory blood pressure measurement used by the Blood Pressure Measurement Laboratory, The Charitable Infirmary, Dublin.

	SBP	DBP	HR			SBP	DBP	HR
No of recordings	45	45	44	Mean of highest five Standard deviation Standard error Coefficient of variation		175·00 12·41 5·55 7·09%	105·40 10·58 4·73 10·03%	94·00 2·53 1·13 2·69%
Peak Trough	196 102	126 61	98 68					
Overall mean Standard deviation Standard error Coefficient of variation	140·16 17·86 2·66 12·74%	85·58 11·57 1·72 13·52%	81·64 7·02 1·06 8·59%	Mean of lowest five Standard deviation Standard error Coefficient of variation		114·40 10·13 4·53 8·86%	67·20 3·54 1·58 5·27%	70·60 1·50 0·67 2·12%

Statistical analysis and plot of 45 ambulatory measurements of blood pressure (systolic and diastolic) and heart rate

Based on a sample page from the *Blood Pressure Booklet*.
(The Blood Pressure Clinic, The Charitable Infirmary, Dublin.)

Assessment of devices for measuring blood pressure

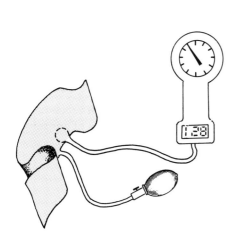

Advances in microcomputer technology are leading inevitably to the marketing of a variety of semiautomated and automated devices for blood pressure measurement. The number of reports on new developments in techniques for measuring blood pressure is surprisingly small, and the reports often lack detail, possibly reflecting the gap between medical and engineering interests. None of the newer devices, no matter how advanced or costly, appears to be better than the simple (and cheap) conventional mercury sphygmomanometers. Worryingly, blood pressure measuring devices may be sold to the public (and to the medical profession) on the basis of claims that have not been assessed adequately. A few independent surveys of semiautomated devices have shown that the standard of engineering and quality control is often poor. Many of these devices are expensive; gadgetry may raise the cost of a sphygmomanometer to above £100 without increasing its accuracy. Ultrasound machines generally cost over £2000, and ambulatory systems may cost in excess of £20000.

Apart from ultrasound techniques, a non-invasive technique superior to Korotkov sound detection with an occluding cuff has not yet been devised for the measurement of blood pressure. Until an alternative method is proved satisfactory all devices are dependent on the cuff occluding technique, and technological advances are restricted to providing automatic cuff inflation and accurate sound detection with a microphone, and to storage and display of the recorded sounds.

Recommendations on blood pressure measurement
Practical points
Explanation to patient
Defence reaction
Variability in blood pressure
Posture of patient
Position of arm
Application of cuff
Position of manometer
Estimation of systolic pressure
Ascultatory measurement of systolic and diastolic pressure
Number of measurements
Indications for measurement in both arms
Times of measurement
Measurement in children
Follow up measurements

For routine clinical measurement of blood pressure in the ward, surgery, or clinic the standard mercury sphygmomanometer and stethoscope is the most economical means of obtaining an accurate measurement of blood pressure. The same is true for the self recording of blood pressures, though if semiautomated devices meeting the requirements for accuracy assessment were available the technique of self measurement would be improved by the removal of observer bias and simplification of the measuring procedure.

In certain circumstances in hospital, such as in theatres and intensive and coronary care units, devices capable of automatic blood pressure measurement and display of data are needed. As the cost of such equipment is high, however, the manufacturers must be able to provide adequate information on accuracy.

Standards for equipment

Points to check in assessing equipment
● *Manometer*—Visibility of meniscus; calibration
● *Cuff*—condition; length and width of inflatable bladder
● *Inflation-deflation device*—possible malfunction; control
● *Stethoscope*—condition
● *Maintenance*—regularity; responsibility

Based on recommendations made by the British Hypertension Society in 1986.

Recommendations on the minimum standards and accuracy requirements for blood pressure measuring devices from official bodies such as the American Association for the Improvement of Medical Instrumentation are to be welcomed. It is time, however, for health authorities in Britain and Ireland to ensure that similar standards are provided by manufacturers. The present unsatisfactory state is that any company may manufacture and market a blood pressure measuring device that claims to be accurate without being required to produce satisfactory information on its accuracy. Some manufacturers do provide evidence of cursory bench accuracy, but few are prepared to subject their equipment to the stringent testing required not only at the time of production but also after a period of time in use. As a result independent laboratories with an interest in blood pressure measurement obtain these devices (usually by paying the full retail price) for testing with the view to publishing the results in one of the medical journals. By the time this is achieved vast sums of money have been spent by hospitals, doctors, and in some cases the public on equipment that may be inaccurate.

This practice should not be allowed to continue. Encouragingly, the British Hypertension Society, which recently published *Recommendations on Blood Pressure Measurement*, is now drawing up guidelines on devices for measuring blood pressure that manufacturers will hopefully enforce so that buyers of equipment will be able to check if the device has an authorised certificate of approval and obtain, on request, the results of accuracy studies.

INDICATIONS FOR TREATMENT

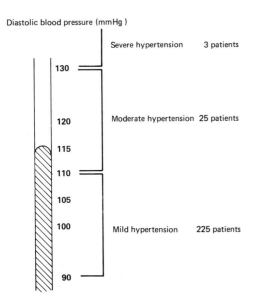

Diastolic blood pressure (mmHg)

Severe hypertension   3 patients

Moderate hypertension 25 patients

Mild hypertension   225 patients

No of patients with raised blood pressure in an average
British general practice (first screening visit, all ages)

Blood pressure has a continuous (bell shaped) distribution in the population—that is, there is no natural dividing line separating normotension from hypertension. Similarly, the risk of complications from hypertension—namely, stroke, myocardial infarction, heart failure, and renal impairment—increases proportionately with rises in blood pressure.

Those at risk

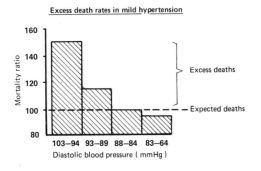

Excess death rates in mild hypertension

Mortality ratio

Excess deaths

Expected deaths

Diastolic blood pressure (mmHg)
103–94 93–89 88–84 83–64

2 year death rate of moderate to severe hypertension

%

Malignant   > 150   149–130 129–120 119–100

Diastolic blood pressure   (mmHg)

On average, a general practitioner with 2500 patients will have three patients with diastolic pressures greater than 130 mm Hg (severe hypertension); if left untreated these patients have a worse prognosis than if they had cancer. Roughly 25 of the general practitioner's patients will have diastolic pressures between 110 and 129 mm Hg (moderate hypertension), and about 20% of these will die in five years. A further 225 patients will have pressures of between 90 and 109 mm Hg (mild hypertension) at first screening, and although many of these pressures fall on retesting, these subjects have a shorter life expectancy than those with pressures that are consistently below this range.

Thus although the personal risk for patients with mild hypertension is much smaller than for those with the severe disease, most heart attacks and strokes occur in those with mild hypertension as there are more people in this category. The epidemiological view is that the whole distribution curve of blood pressure in Western countries is too high, and a downward shift of no more than 5 mm Hg in the average pressure of the population would improve the average life expectancy dramatically.

Contrary to popular belief, systolic pressure is a better predictor of risk than diastolic pressure. Patients with isolated systolic hypertension (systolic pressure above 160 mm Hg and diastolic pressure below 90 mm Hg) also have an increased risk of stroke and myocardial infarction.

Benefits of treatment

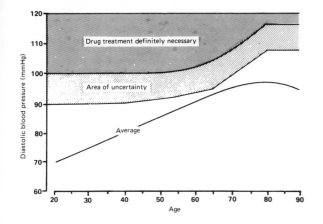

The absence of a natural threshold blood pressure that defines hypertension produces the dilemma of when to start treatment. A practical definition of hypertension, provided by Rose, is the level of blood pressure "at which the benefits . . . of action exceed those of inaction."

During the past 20 years a series of clinical trials have attempted to define the lowest limit of blood pressure above which treatment is of benefit. For patients aged under 70 diastolic pressures consistently above 100 mm Hg are an indication for treatment, implying that diastolic pressure should be reduced below this level. Reduction to below 90 mm Hg may be of value in preventing stroke, but large numbers have to be treated for the benefit of a few. A more aggressive policy might be used for those patients with evidence of damage to target organs—that is, retinopathy, left ventricular hypertrophy, and renal failure—or a strong family history of premature death from hypertensive complications.

The benefits of lowering systolic pressure have received little attention in the major clinical trials. Systolic pressure is more difficult to reduce to satisfactory levels than diastolic pressure, but a systolic pressure of below 160 mm Hg for most patients aged under 70 and below 140 mm Hg for those under 40 should be attempted.

Unless the blood pressure is particularly high (diastolic blood pressure >110 mm Hg) or there is evidence of damage to target organs, several recordings over four to six weeks should be made, with the patient relaxed, before a decision to treat is taken.

Balancing risks and benefits

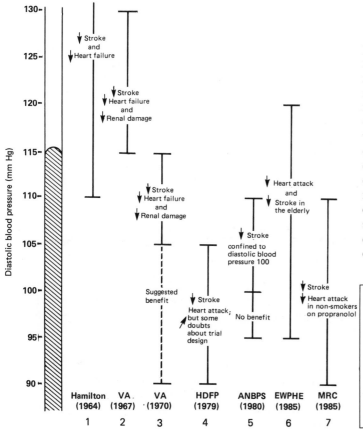

Hypertension does not generally cause any symptoms. On the other hand, treatment, even non-pharmacological treatment, has its drawbacks. A balance has to be struck between the benefits of long term treatment and its inconveniences. The benefits are the hoped for prolongation of life with freedom from stroke, heart failure, and renal complications and possibly a lowered risk of heart attack. These must be weighed against the repeated visits to the surgery, numerous blood pressure readings, initial blood tests and other investigations, the chore of taking tablets every day, and the side effects of the tablets. An explanation of the problem and the expectations from treatment in terms that the patient can understand is important to allay anxiety and encourage compliance. Poor compliance with treatment is a major potential stumbling block in the management of each patient's blood pressure, and time spent at this stage is repaid in the succeeding decades of care. The doctor must, however, avoid inducing hypochondria caused by diagnosis and treatment.

References
1 Hamilton M, Thompson EN, Wisniewski TKM. *Lancet*, 1964; i: 235–8.
2 Veterans Administration Co-operative Study Group on Antihypertensive Agents. *JAMA* 1967, 202: 1028–34.
3 Veterans Administration Co-operative Study Group on Antihypertensive Agents. *JAMA* 1970; 213: 1143–52.
4 Hypertension Detection and Follow-up Program Cooperative Group. The effect of treatment on mortality in "mild hypertension". *N Engl J Med* 1982; 307: 976–80.
5 Australian National Blood Pressure Study Management Committee. The Australian therapeutic trial in mild hypertension. *Lancet* 1980; ii: 1261–6.
6 Amery A, Birkenhager W, Brixho P, *et al.* Mortality and morbidity results from the European Working Party on High Blood Pressure in the Elderly trial. *Lancet* 1985; i: 1349–54.
7 Medical Research Council Working Party, MRC trial of mild hypertension, principal results. *Br Med J* 1985; 291: 104.

NON-PHARMACOLOGICAL MANAGEMENT

In addition to noting damage to target organs and coexisting disease, the doctor should assess the patient's lifestyle. Other risk factors for atheroma, such as cigarette smoking, may be identified while advice on weight reduction and salt and alcohol intake may be indicated. Such measures are additive to pharmacological treatment and may be all that is necessary for some patients with mild hypertension. Indeed, in the light of the Medical Research Council trial in 1985 on the drug treatment of mild hypertension non-pharmacological management should assume much greater importance.

Obesity

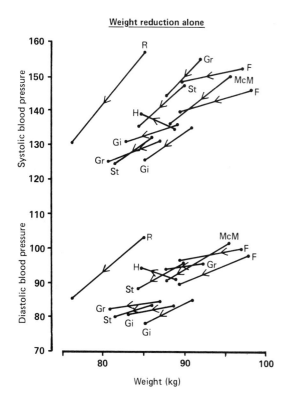

Weight reduction alone

Obesity is strongly associated with hypertension. Several but not all studies have shown a reduction in systolic and diastolic pressures with weight loss (figure). A reduction in weight of 3 kg produces an estimated fall in blood pressure of 7/4 mm Hg; a weight loss of 12 kg gives a fall of 21/13 mm Hg. Every attempt should be made to get obese patients to diet so that their weight falls within the norm for their height and build. It is worth while providing patients with diet sheets or referring them to a dietitian.

References
F: Fagenberg B, Andersson OV, Isaksson B, Björntorp P. *Br Med J* 1984; **288:** 11–14.
Gi: 6 Gillum RF, Prineas RF, Jeffery RW, *et al. Am Heart J* 1983; 105; **128:** 32.
GR: Greminger P, Studer A, Lüscher T *et al. Schweiz Med Wochenschr* 1982 112: 120–4.
H: Haynes RO, Harper AC, Costley SR, *et al.* J Hypertension 1984; 2: 535–9.
McM: MacMahon S, MacDonald GJ, Berstein L, *et al. Lancet* 1985; i: 1233–6.
R: Reisin E, Abel R, Modan M, *et al. N Engl J Med* 1978; **298:** 1–6.
St: Stamler J, Farinaro E, Mojonnier LM, *et al. JAMA* 1980; **243:** 1819–23.

Salt

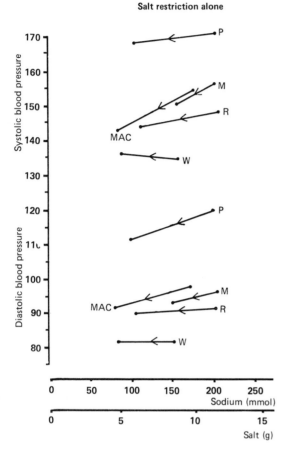

Salt restriction alone

Change in blood pressure with salt restriction alone
(each line represents one published study)

Severe reduction in the intake of salt (10 mmol/day) reduces blood pressure but also renders the diet unpalatable. Controversy surrounds the value of moderate restriction in the intake of salt (60 to 80 mmol/day), but some studies have shown this to be helpful (figure); it may be achieved by not adding salt to food after cooking and avoiding heavily salted "convenience" foods like hamburgers, sausages, and salty bacon. Many patients find this acceptable, and it is certainly not harmful.

References
M: Morgan T, Adam W, Gillies A, et al. Lancet 1978; i: 227–30.
MAC: GA MacGregor, ND Markand, FE Best et al. Lancet 1982; **1:** 351–5.
P: Parijis J, Joosens JV, Van der Linden L, Verstreken, Amery A Am Heart J 1973; **85:** 22–34.
R: Richards AM, Nicholls MG, Espine EAP, et al. Lancet 1984; i: 757–61.
W: Watt GCM, Edwards C, Hart JT, Hart M, Walton P, Foy CJW. Br Med J 1983; **286:** 432–6.

Alcohol

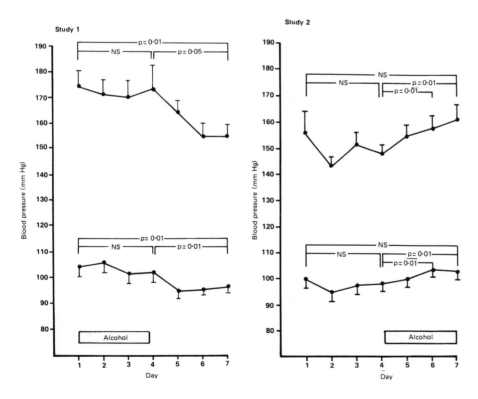

An association between alcohol intake and hypertension is well noted in both population and clinical studies. An alcohol intake of around 80 g alcohol/day (equivalent to four pints of beer) has been shown to raise blood pressure, particularly in hypertensive patients; blood pressure falls soon after stopping drinking and remains low in those who continue to abstain. All hypertensive patients should be encouraged to reduce their alcohol intake to an average of no more than two drinks a day. One "drink" is equivalent to one glass of wine or sherry, one tot of spirits, or half a pint of beer. The figures show the changes seen in blood pressure in untreated hypertensive patients when they stop drinking (study 1) or when they restart their alcohol intake (study 2).

From Potters JF, Beevers DG. Lancet 1984; i: 119–22.

Non-pharmacological management

Cigarette smoking

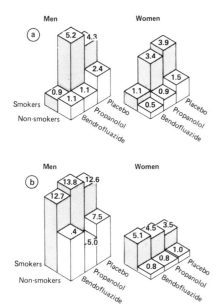

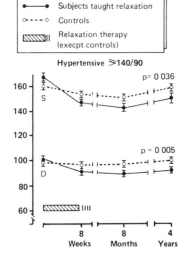

(a) Incidence of stroke per 1000 patient years

(b) Incidence of coronary disease per 1000 patient years

There is a strong association between cigarette smoking and malignant hypertension. Furthermore, smoking induces hepatic enzymes, and there is evidence that smokers respond less well to some antihypertensive drugs, notably those β blockers that are cleared by hepatic metabolism. For these reasons, and because cigarette smoking is an independent risk factor for vascular disease, hypertensive patients should be persuaded to stop smoking completely.

The MRC Working Party on Hypertension. *Br Med J* 1985 291: 102.

Relaxation therapy

Reports on the effects of behavioural therapy on blood pressure have been encouraging: treatment of this type for eight weeks has been shown to produce a sustained fall in blood pressure for as long as one year. It requires, however, motivated patients.

From Patel R, Marmot MG, Terry DJ, Curuthers M, Hunt B, Patel M. *Br Med J* 1985; **290:** 1126.

Hypertension induced by drugs

1 Drugs causing sodium retention: oral corticosteroids, ACTH, liquorice, carbenoxolone, phenylbutazone, indomethacin

2 Drugs causing increased sympathomimetic activity: ephedrine, cold cures, monoamine oxidase inhibitors

3 Direct vasoconstrictors: ergot alkaloids

4 Oral contraceptives, oestrogen therapy

5 Drug withdrawal - clonidine

6 Interactions with antihypertensive drugs: tricyclic antidepressants, indomethacin

Blood pressure almost invariably rises in women taking the oral contraceptive, but usually the rise is too small to be clinically important.

In about 5% of women diastolic pressures rise above 90 mm Hg. In some cases pressures may fall if a progestagen only pill is used. Other methods of contraception should be used if blood pressures do not settle.

DRUG TREATMENT I: FIRST CHOICE AGENTS

The traditional approach to the drug treatment of hypertension has been step care, in which treatment began with a β blocker or thiazide and progressed to a combination of the two, followed, in more resistant patients, by the addition of a vasodilator. Over the past five years two new classes of cardiovascular drugs, the calcium antagonists and the angiotensin converting enzyme inhibitors, have challenged this rigid approach. Although β blockers and thiazides remain popular choices, the newer drugs are effective, and, used with care, they are well tolerated and are suitable for use as first line agents. The broader range of drugs now available gives greater facility for the choice to be tailored to the patient's individual circumstances.

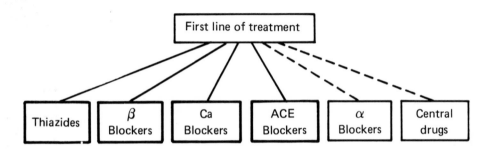

Thiazide diuretics

Recommended for:	Older patients
	Black patients
	Patients with heart failure (mild)
Avoid in:	Maturity onset diabetics
	Hyperuricaemic patients
Side effects:	Hypokalaemia
	Hyperuricaemia
	Hyperglycaemia
	Impotence
	Rashes
	Blood dyscrasias

Thiazide diuretics are still of value in the treatment of hypertension. They are cheap, effective, easy to use, and can be given once daily. They are well absorbed from the gut and are excreted through the kidney.

Blood pressure is lowered by a combination of increased excretion of renal sodium and water, thereby reducing blood volume, and a direct effect of the drugs on vascular smooth muscle, reducing peripheral vascular resistance. The dose response curve with respect to blood pressure is flat—that is, increasing the dose beyond a certain threshold has little further hypotensive effect. In contrast, the risks of hypokalaemia and probably hyperuricaemia and hyperglycaemia continue to increase. Lower doses are therefore recommended (bendrofluazide 2·5 mg, hydrochlorthiazide 25 mg) than have been prescribed in the past.

Hypokalaemia is more common in patients treated with thiazide diuretics than loop diuretics. The risks of mild hypokalaemia (potassium concentration 3·0–3·5 mmol/l) continue to be debated. We recommend correcting hypokalaemia, if it occurs, with potassium sparing diuretics, or changing to another first line drug.

The loop diuretics such as frusemide are less potent as antihypertensive agents but are indicated when there is concomitant cardiac or renal failure (thiazides are less effective when there is renal impairment) and in resistant hypertension, when fluid retention due to other antihypertensive drugs may contribute to the raised blood pressure.

Drug treatment I: first choice agents

β blockers

Recommended for:	Young patients Anxious patients Patients with concomitant angina Patients who have had a myocardial infarction Non-smokers
Avoid in:	Asthma Heart failure Heart block Peripheral disease Brittle insulin dependent diabetes
Side effects:	Bronchospasm Impaired response Negative intropy to hypoglycaemia Bradycardia Hyperlipidaemia Cold hands and feet Hyperuricaemia Fatigue Vivid dreams

Beta blockers competitively inhibit the action of catecholamines on β adrenoceptors. Some block both β_1 receptors (heart rate and contractility) and β_2 receptors (vascular and bronchial smooth muscle), whereas others block mainly β_1 receptors and are fairly cardioselective. Used carefully, they are effective and safe. They are well absorbed from the gastrointestinal tract. Some are metabolised in the liver; some are excreted renally and the dose of these should be reduced in patients with renal failure; others are excreted by both routes. Beta blockers are thought to lower blood pressure by reducing cardiac output and having a central effect on the vasomotor centre. As with thiazide diuretics, β blockers show a flat dose blood pressure response curve; there is little value in increasing the dose above that recommended, though higher doses may be tried in black patients who are thought to be less responsive to β blockers. If blood pressure is not reduced by one β blocker it is unlikely to be reduced by changing to another. The choice of β blocker depends on other properties of these drugs.

Pharmacological properties of some blockers

	Relative cardioselectivity	Partial agonist activity	Lipophilic (L)* or hydrophilic (H)	Renal (R) or hepatic (H) elimination
Acebutolol	+	+	L	H (active metabolite R)
Atenolol	++	−	H	R
Metoprolol	++	−	L	H
Nadolol	−	−	H	R
Oxprenolol	−	+	L	H
Pindolol	−	++	L	H
Propranolol	−	−	L	H
Sotalol	−	−	H	R
Timolol	−	−	L	H

*Lipophilicity—hydrophilicity represent a spectrum; propranolol is very lipophilic; atenolol, nadolol, sotalol are hydrophilic; and the others occupy an intermediate position.

The lipophilic β blockers are more likely to have side effects on the central nervous system; the water soluble drugs are excreted renally and have longer half lives and can be given once daily. The cardioselective β blockers are less likely to aggravate peripheral vascular disease or impair diabetic control. Partial agonist activity is associated with less resting bradycardia and is of theoretical value in patients complaining of cold hands and feet or peripheral ischaemia.

All β blockers are contraindicated in patients with a history of wheeze. Beware of β blockers hidden in combination preparations in which the name does not suggest the inclusion of a β blocker.

Calcium antagonists

Recommended for:	Asthmatic patients Patients with concomitant angina Patients with peripheral vascular disease
Avoid in:	Verapamil and diltiazem are contraindicated in patients with heart block Use with care with digoxin and β blockers
Side effects:	Flushing Headache Ankle swelling Gum hyperplasia

Calcium antagonists are a chemically heterogeneous group, to which more drugs are being added. They inhibit the transport of calcium ions across cell membranes. The transport of calcium ions is important for generating action potentials and for muscle contraction. These drugs reduce blood pressure by vasodilatation. The three calcium antagonists currently available—nifedipine, verapamil, diltiazem—differ in affinity for cardiac conducting tissue (slowing atrioventricular nodal conduction), cardiac muscle (reducing contractility), and vascular smooth muscle (peripheral vasodilatation). Nifedipine (20–40 mg twice daily) has little effect on the atrioventricular node but is a potent vasodilator. Verapamil (120 mg twice daily) is a useful antiarrhythmic drug with some vasodilatory action. Diltiazem (60 mg thrice daily) has some effect on both cardiac conduction and vascular smooth muscle. All are well absorbed from the gastrointestinal tract and undergo first pass metabolism in the liver.

	Nifedipine	Verapamil	Diltiazem	Nicardipine
Vascular smooth muscle	+++	+	++	++
Atrio-ventricular node	−	+++	++	−
Cardiac muscle	+	+	−	−

Verapamil and diltiazem are contraindicated in patients with heart block and should be used with care in patients taking digoxin or β blockers because of the additive effect on nodal conduction. They also increase plasma concentrations of digoxin. The side effects of nifedipine and diltiazem are headache and flushing, which may tend to improve with continued use. Ankle oedema is thought to be due to a direct effect of these drugs on capillary permeability and is not responsive to diuretics.

Angiotensin converting enzyme inhibitors

Recommended for:	Heart failure (but care with diuretics)
	Peripheral vascular disease
Caution with:	Chronic renal disease when used with potassium sparing diuretics and non-steroidal anti-inflammatory drugs
Avoid in:	Bilateral renal artery stenosis in fluid depleted patients
Side effects:	Taste disturbance
	Cough
	Hypotension in volume depleted patients
	Rashes
	Neutropenia
	Proteinuria
	Angioneurotic oedema

Angiotensin converting enzyme is responsible for converting angiotensin I to angiotensin II (a potent vasoconstrictor and stimulator of aldosterone secretion) and for the breakdown of bradykinin (a vasodilator). The angiotensin converting enzyme inhibitors captopril and enalapril lower blood pressure by reducing peripheral vascular resistance and, to a lesser extent, by preventing reabsorption of sodium by aldosterone. Enalapril is an ester of the active compound and is activated by hydrolysis in the liver. It is a more potent angiotensin converting enzyme inhibitor than captopril and can be given once daily. Both are well tolerated in uncomplicated hypertension, but they should be used with care in the elderly and in patients with renal impairment (because renal function may deteriorate) and in patients taking diuretics (to avoid precipitous falls in blood pressure). Treatment should be introduced in low doses (captopril 12.5 mg twice daily, enalapril 5 mg daily—or 2·5 mg for patients over 65 years, patients with renal impairment, and when used with diuretics), and thereafter the dose should be increased gradually. For patients with normal renal function, the dose should not exceed 150 mg daily for captopril, 40 mg daily for enalapril.

The side effects of captopril were attributed initially to its sulphahydryl group, but this is no longer thought to be true. Enalapril, which does not have this chemical group, seems to have a similar profile of side effects. The incidence of rashes seems to depend on dose. Disturbance in taste is usually transitory and resolves with continued treatment. The frequency of neutropenia increases if renal function is impaired and when it occurs it does so almost invariably in the first three months. Cough may disappear with time or a reduction in dose, but it may persist and require different drug treatment in some patients. Proteinuria may occur, and nephrotic syndrome has been reported in patients treated with captopril, but the loss of protein usually decreases with time even when treatment is continued.

Other suitable drugs

Recommended in:	Asthmatic patients
	Patients with peripheral vascular disease
	Patients with heart failure
Side effects:	First dose syncope
	Sedation
	Fluid retention
	Dry mouth

Prazosin is an α blocker; it antagonises the stimulation of vascular α_1 receptors and dilates both arterial and venous blood vessels. It reduces peripheral vascular resistance without inducing a reflex tachycardia and is well absorbed after being given orally, but has to be given two to three times a day. The initial dose should be low as it can cause a precipitous fall in blood pressure and syncope. Starter packs are available, and it is usual to give the first dose (0·5 mg) to the patient in bed at night. Thereafter the dose may be increased (avoiding sharp increases) to a maximum of 30 mg daily in divided doses. The hypotensive effect may be enhanced by adding a thiazide diuretic. If treatment is introduced gradually the drug is usually well tolerated.

Can be tried in:	Asthmatic patients
	Patients with heart failure
	Patients with claudication
	Diabetes
Avoid in:	Depression
	Liver disease
Side effects:	Hepatitis
	Haemolytic anaemia
	Sedation
	Dry mouth
	Impotence

Methyldopa is still used widely in the treatment of hypertension. Its mechanism of action is not fully understood, but it is thought to act on the central nervous system to reduce sympathetic outflow. Its major disadvantages are that it needs to be given thrice daily and produces a high incidence of side effects when large doses (1 g thrice daily) are required. The usual dose is 250–500 mg thrice daily, and its therapeutic effect may be enhanced by combination with a diuretic. The drug is excreted by the kidney and so a reduction in dose may be necessary in patients with renal failure.

DRUG TREATMENT II: COMBINATION TREATMENT, RESISTANT HYPERTENSION, ALTERNATIVE DRUGS

Combination treatment

		Add if no contraindications					
		T	BB	N	V	ACE	P
First choice drug is	Thiazide (T)	–	1	2	2	2	2
	β blocker (BB)	1	–	2	✗	2	2
	Nifedipine (N)	2	1	–	–	2	
	Verapamil (V)	1	✗	–	–		
	Angiotensin converting (ACE) enzyme inhibitor	1	2	2		–	
	Prazosin (P)	1	2				–

1= First preference	☐ Benefit unassessed		
2= Alternatives	✗ Don't do		

Although the number of drugs available for treating hypertension has increased, the underlying principles of treatment have not changed. The concept of step care remains: drug treatment is started with one agent and other drugs (from different classes) are added "step wise," until satisfactory control is achieved. At the same time treatment should always be kept as simple as possible to aid compliance.

If the first drug chosen does not lead to a satisfactory fall in blood pressure there may be room to increase the dose. This may be helpful when using prazosin, a calcium antagonist, or angiotensin converting enzyme inhibitor. The next step is to add a second drug. The flowchart gives some suggestions for combinations of drugs. The choice of second drug should again be tailored to the patient—for example, a diuretic should be given if there is fluid retention. When tolerated, the combination of a β blocker and a diuretic remains useful as they may be prescribed in a combination tablet, thereby reducing the daily intake of tablets.

Hypertension in most patients is controlled by one or two drugs. If blood pressure is not adequately reduced it is worth checking to see that the patient is actually taking the tablets. If drug compliance is not a problem the next step is to add a third drug. Most combinations are suitable but the following should be avoided: verapamil and β blockers; two drugs from the same class.

Resistant hypertension

1. Are tablets being taken ?

2. Are side effects preventing adherence ?

3. Check again for underlying cause

If diastolic blood pressure is still over 110 mm Hg despite triple dose treatment consideration should be given to: compliance; secondary hypertension. These patients are probably best managed in hospital clinics.

When essential hypertension is genuinely resistant to treatment, the substitution of frusemide for the thiazide diuretic may further reduce blood pressure.

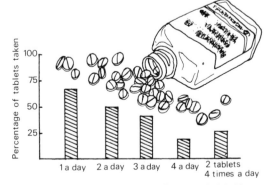

From Gatley MS. *J R Coll Gen Pract* 1968; **16:** 39.

Another approach is to use minoxidil. This drug has a direct effect on arteries by causing vasodilatation; it does not dilate veins. Side effects are common and so it is reserved for patients with resistant hypertension. Fluid retention and tachycardia mean that it must be used in conjunction with a diuretic and a β blocker. Hypertrichosis occurs after about three weeks of treatment: it is reversible but may be cosmetically unacceptable to women. T wave changes (flattening or inversion) in the electrocardiograph are common within a few days of starting minoxidil but usually resolve with continued treatment.

Some patients require four antihypertensive drugs, but the best combination has yet to be found by trial.

Drug treatment II: combination treatment, resistant hypertension, alternative drugs

Alternative antihypertensive drugs

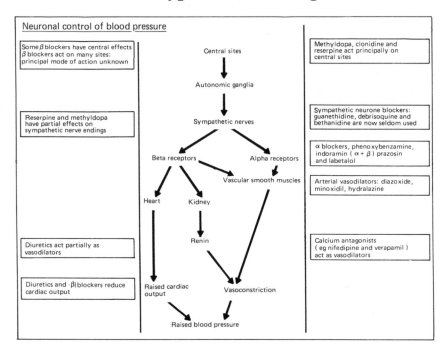

Hydralazine is a direct acting vasodilator—primarily on the arterial circulation. It is well absorbed after being taken by mouth. It may also be given by intravenous or intramuscular injection. Hydralazine is extensively metabolised in the liver by acetylation and must be given at least twice daily. The population can be divided into two groups, "slow acetylators" and "fast acetylators". The slow acetylators are thought to be more susceptible to developing a syndrome resembling systemic lupus erythematosus and a rheumatoid like arthropathy. These syndromes are more common when doses exceeding 200 mg a day are used but they may also occur with lower doses, particularly in patients who are slow acetylators. Combination treatment with a β blocker and a diuretic is required to counteract reflex tachycardia and fluid retention. Other side effects include headache and nasal congestion.

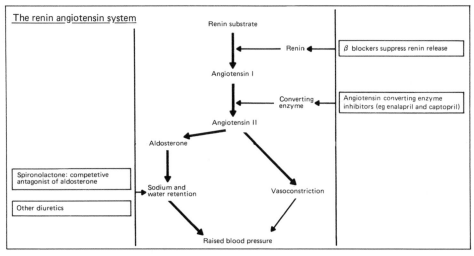

Sites of action of antihypertensive drugs

Other useful drugs include the diuretics spironolactone, amiloride, and triampterene. Spironolactone is metabolised to canterone, which acts as an aldosterone antagonist. It is a mild diuretic, with potassium retaining properties. It is used to treat Conn's syndrome but is also prescribed with other diuretics to reduce loss of potassium. In patients with renal failure it can cause hyperkalaemia. Side effects include gynaecomastia, menstrual disturbances, and peptic ulceration.

Amiloride and triampterene are diuretics that also retain potassium, and these are used mainly in conjunction with other diuretics to reduce potassium loss. They produce few side effects but hyperkalaemia may occur. They should not be prescribed with angiotensin converting enzyme inhibitors.

Other α blockers include indoramin, a selective α₁ adrenoceptor antagonist similar to prazosin, which acts as a vasodilator with little reflex tachycardia. The initial dose is 25 mg twice daily, and the dose is gradually increased (every two weeks), according to response, to a maximum of 100 mg twice daily. Sedation is dose related. Other reported side effects are depression, dizziness, dry mouth, and nasal congestion. It should not be prescribed with monoamine oxidase (MAD) inhibitors.

Phenoxybenzamine is a non-selective α blocker used primarily to treat hypertension secondary to phaeochromocytoma. Side effects include sedation, postural hypotension, failure to ejaculate, and nasal congestion.

Labetalol is a combined α and β blocking agent, combining the benefits of reducing peripheral resistance with those of β blockade. It may be given intravenously in hypertensive emergencies and perioperatively in the management of phaechromocytoma. The contraindications are the same as those of β blockers.

SPECIAL PROBLEMS

Diabetes mellitus

Recommended:	Angiotensin converting enzyme inhibitors
	Prazosin
	Hydralazine
	Methyldopa
	(Calcium antagonists)
Caution:	β blockers
	Thiazides

Diabetes mellitus and hypertension often occur together: although obesity is a factor common to both conditions, this does not completely explain the association. Raised blood pressure accelerates the cardiovascular and renal complications associated with raised blood glucose concentration. Adequate treatment of coexisting hypertension delays the development of these complications.

When obesity is present, blood pressure may improve with a reduction in weight. When drug treatment is necessary, care has to be taken over the choice of agent used. Chronic treatment with thiazide diuretics impairs glucose tolerance and cannot be recommended for diabetic patients being treated with carbohydrate restriction or oral hypoglycaemic agents. These may, however, be used in insulin dependent diabetes as any further impairment of glucose tolerance can be compensated for by a small increase in the dose of insulin.

Beta blockers may impair the metabolic response to hypoglycaemia. Although in theory this is less likely using the cardioselective agents metoprolol and atenolol, all β blockers are best avoided in brittle diabetes; but these are safe in most patients receiving insulin. β blockers should be avoided in diabetics with peripheral arterial disease.

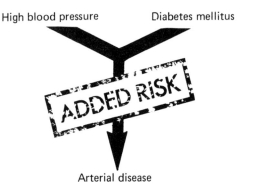

High blood pressure   Diabetes mellitus

Arterial disease

In theory calcium antagonists may impair insulin release and consequently glucose tolerance, but current evidence does not substantiate this.

The angiotensin converting enzyme inhibitors prazosin and methyldopa may be used safely and are the drugs of choice for hypertensive diabetic patients.

Heart failure

Recommended:	Diuretics
	Calcium antagonists
	Angiotensin converting enzyme inhibitors
	Prazosin
	Methyldopa
Avoid with:	β blockers
	Verapamil

Hypertension may cause heart failure, which may be the presenting problem. Beta blockers reduce cardiac output and may provoke or aggravate heart failure. To a lesser degree some calcium antagonists are also negative inotropes, and this may outweigh any beneficial effect to be derived from their vasodilatory action. They should be used cautiously in patients with heart failure.

Diuretics are a logical first line treatment. Depending on the severity of heart failure, a loop acting diuretic, such as frusemide, may be necessary.

The angiotensin converting enzyme inhibitors are also favoured as they are used in the treatment of heart failure. In addition to vasodilatation, the action of these drugs on the renin-angiotensin-aldosterone axis also helps reduce fluid retention. They must be introduced with care, however, starting at a low dose and gradually increasing, to avoid a precipitous fall in blood pressure. Prazosin and methyldopa are safe and may be usefully added to diuretic treatment.

Ischaemic heart disease

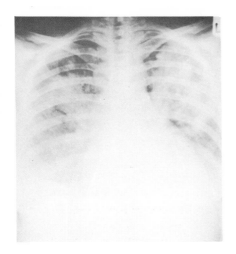

Recommended	β blockers
	Calcium antagonists

Obstructive airways disease

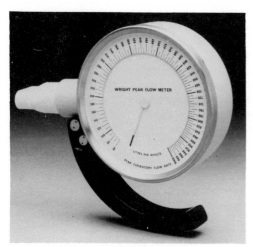

The photograph of the Wright Peak Flow Meter is produced by kind permission of Clement Clarke International Limited.

Renal failure

Recommended:	Loop diuretics (except ethacrynic acid)
	β blockers
	Calcium antagonists
	Prazosin
	Methyldopa
Caution:	Angiotensin converting enzyme inhibitors

In patients with hypertension and angina symptoms may be alleviated if their blood pressure is reduced by any drug. Beta blockers and calcium antagonists, however, have specific antianginal actions and convey added advantages, so they are the drugs of choice. Furthermore, increasing evidence suggests that β blockers given at the time of or soon after myocardial infarction may help to reduce the occurrence of a second infarct. Care must be taken to observe the contraindications to β blockade—namely, bradyarrhythmias and heart failure—which are associated with myocardial infarction. Verapamil should be used cautiously with a β blocker, but nifedipine is quite safe.

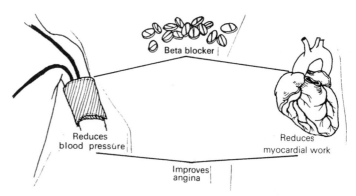

Beta blockers cannot be recommended for any patient with wheeze or a history of wheeze. Even cardioselective (β_1 receptor blocking) drugs are not completely safe for two reasons: firstly, there are some β_1 receptors in bronchial smooth muscle; secondly, selectivity is relative, and some cross interaction with β_2 receptors occurs when high plasma concentrations of these drugs are achieved.

In contrast, the calcium antagonists may confer a degree of protection against bronchospasm in patients with a history of asthma. Although the benefit shown to date is small, it nevertheless favours the use of calcium antagonists as the drugs of choice for hypertensive patients with coexisting obstructive airways disease.

Recommended:	Diuretics
	Calcium antagonists
	Angiotensin converting enzyme inhibitors
	Prazosin
	Hydralazine
	Methyldopa
Avoid:	β blockers

Good control of blood pressure is essential in patients with chronic renal failure to prevent further deterioration in renal function. At the same time care must also be taken to avoid hypotension and a critical reduction in renal blood flow. Treatment may include dietary salt restriction (to 100 mmol/day) and often large doses of a loop diuretic (not ethacrynic acid because of the risk of deafness) to prevent fluid retention. If the blood pressure remains high a β blocker or calcium antagonist can be added. These drugs are much favoured in renal failure, although prazosin or methyldopa can also be used.

Special problems

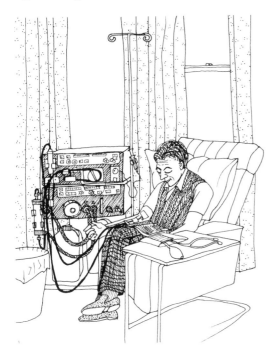

Some patients will have "resistant hypertension" and will require more than one drug. Others, particularly those with severe renal impairment (glomerular filtration rate < 10 ml/minute), are extremely sensitive to hypotensive drugs. Furthermore, some of the β blockers—for example, atenolol, nadolol, and sotalol—are excreted in the urine and accumulate in renal failure. If possible all hypotensive drugs should be introduced in low doses and the dose gradually increased to achieve the desired effect. Regular monitoring of serum creatinine concentration and electrolytes, as well as blood pressure, are necessary to assess response to treatment.

The angiotensin converting enzyme inhibitors should be used with particular care. Blood pressure may fall precipitously at the start of treatment with these drugs, and reports of deteriorating renal function associated with their use have emerged .

Once the patient has started dialysis, blood pressure is usually easily controlled by the removal of salt and water.

After a stroke

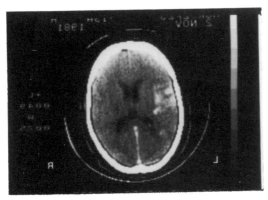

In patients under 65 years who have had a stroke and whose diastolic pressure is greater than 105 mm Hg antihypertensive treatment definitely helps to prevent a second stroke. Nevertheless, because cerebral autoregulation of blood flow is disturbed immediately after a stroke, treatment should be started only during the recovery phase or when the patient is attending an outpatient follow up clinic. Sudden drops in blood pressure should be avoided, so that drugs that cause postural hypotension (bethanicline, debrisoquine, and guanethidine) should not be used.

The value of treating hypertension in the elderly before or after a stroke is unproved. Treatment should therefore be less aggressive.

Depression

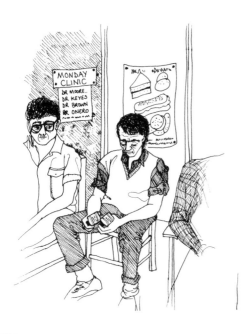

Recommended:
Thiazide diuretics
Calcium antagonists
Angiotensin converting enzyme inhibitors
Avoid:
Methyldopa
Reserpine

Although no association exists between hypertension as a disease and depression, depression may be a side effect of treatment. Methyldopa, reserpine, and the rauwolfia alkaloids are well recognised causes of depression. Beta blockers may cause lethargy and fatigue. The angiotensin converting enzyme inhibitors seem to cause fewer side effects on the central nervous system than other drugs.

Impotence

```
┌─────────────────────────────────────────┐
│                                           │
│   Recommended:                            │
│         Thiazide diuretics                │
│         Calcium antagonists               │
│         Angiotensin converting enzyme     │
│         inhibitors                        │
│                                           │
│   Avoid:                                  │
│         Methyldopa                        │
│         Reserpine                         │
│                                           │
└─────────────────────────────────────────┘
```

Some hypotensive drugs induce impotence and while other causes, such as alcoholism, diabetes mellitus, and psychiatric disorders, should be considered, it is wise to avoid those drugs that have been associated with this problem. In the Medical Research Council trial of mild hypertension impotence was found to be more common in the subgroup receiving thiazide diuretics than in the group receiving placeboes. Methyldopa, hydralazine, and β blockers are also thought to induce impotence.

EMERGENCY REDUCTION IN BLOOD PRESSURE: MALIGNANT HYPERTENSION

The diagnosis of malignant hypertension is made on the basis of very high blood pressure (diastolic blood pressures usually more than 130 mm Hg), together with retinal haemorrhages, and exudates with or without papilloedema. Similar high blood pressures without these fundal changes may be seen. Although some patients may be severely ill with heart failure or occasionally encephalopathy at presentation, most are remarkably well or complain only of blurring of vision or headache. The prognosis for all patients with untreated severe hypertension, however, is so poor that urgent treatment, preferably with admission to hospital, is essential.

Diagnosis:

- Diastolic blood pressure >130 mmHg

- Retinal haemorrhages

- Exudates with or without papilloedema

Indications for parenteral antihypertensive drugs

Indications for parenteral antihypertensive drugs

There are very few indications
Gross ventricular failure due to hypertension
Encephalopathy with fits or fluctuating neurological signs
Eclampsia with fits
Control of blood pressure in managing aortic dissection

Parenteral antihypertensive treatment

1	Labetalol	40–80 mg/hour by infusion
2	Nitroprusside	0·5–8 µg/kg/minute
3	Diazoxide	50 mg mini bolus injection repeat as necessary
4	Hydralazine	5–20 mg intramuscularly or intravenously

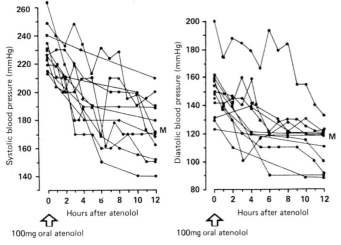

Effects of single oral dose of atenolol in severe hypertension

(Case M was given a second 100mg dose after 4½ hours)

The hazards of very rapid reduction in blood pressure include stroke, blindness, and myocardial infarction: the aim should be to reduce gradually the diastolic pressure over several hours. This can usually be achieved with bed rest and drug treatment by mouth. Malignant hypertension is not itself an indication for parenteral treatment.

From Bannan LT, Beevers DG. *Drugs* 1983; **25** (suppl 3): 84.

Patients without heart failure or encephalopathy

Recommended:

> β blocker (including labetalol)
> Nifedipine
> Methyldopa
> Hydralazine

Avoid:

> Prazosin
> Angiotensin converting enzyme
> inhibitors

A modest fall in blood pressure may occur with bed rest. If there is no contraindication, such as asthma, a β blocker such as atenolol (50 or 100 mg) is recommended. When β blockers cannot be used, nifedipine 10 to 20 mg, methyldopa 250 mg, or hydralazine 25 mg are suitable alternatives. Beta blockers should not be used alone in patients in whom phaeochromocytoma is suspected. Pending confirmation of the diagnosis, the addition of an α blocker is required, such as can be provided by phenoxybenzamine or labetalol 100–200 mg.

In general, diuretics are of little value, except where there is evidence of pulmonary oedema, when a loop diuretic such as frusemide should be given.

If a single dose of antihypertensive drug does not reduce blood pressure within four hours a further dose can be given by mouth. The objective should be to reduce the diastolic pressure to about 110 mm Hg over the first 12 hours. Perfect control of blood pressure, which usually requires the administration of two or more drugs, should be sought over the next few days.

Patients with heart failure

Recommended initially:

> Nitroprusside, or diamorphine
> and frusemide

Secondarily:

> Diuretics
> Calcium antagonists
> Prazosin

If there is severe left ventricular failure associated with a diastolic blood pressure over 140 mm Hg the drug of choice is sodium nitroprusside. This is given by intravenous infusion in a dose of 0·5 µg/kg/minute, increasing, if necessary, to 8 µg/kg/minute. (Nitroprusside powder (50 mg) is dissolved in 1 litre of 5% dextrose and covered with reflective foil to prevent photodegradation. About 100–200 ml of this solution is usually given over one hour.) Response should be monitored by measuring blood pressure every 60 seconds and the infusion rate adjusted to avoid dropping the diastolic blood pressure lower than 100–110 mm Hg. Fresh nitroprusside solutions have to be made every four hours. Treatment by mouth should be started as soon as possible, and more than one drug is usually required. Suddenly stopping the nitroprusside infusion may lead to a sudden rise in blood pressure if oral treatment is not effective. The infusion should be gradually decreased as the oral treatment takes effect.

Patients with encephalopathy

Recommended:

> Nitroprusside
> Labetalol

Hypertensive encephalopathy is rare. The diagnosis is difficult, and more often than not any neurological deficit in a patient with severe hypertension is due to cerebral infarction or haemorrhage. Cerebral infarction and haemorrhage are specific contraindications to the rapid reduction in blood pressure, as this may worsen the neurological deficit. Encephalopathy is more likely if there are convulsions, fluctuating levels of consciousness, or fluctuating neurological signs.

Sodium nitroprusside by infusion, as previously described, is the treatment of choice because of the fine control it gives over reduction in blood pressure. An alternative drug is labetalol (1–3 mg/minute by intravenous infusion).

THE ELDERLY

The problem

In most societies blood pressure rises with age, at least until the age of 70, when average diastolic blood pressure falls but systolic pressure continues to rise. In developed countries findings based on a single casual blood pressure reading over 160/95 mm Hg show that the prevalence of hypertension approaches 50% in patients over 70 years, with a further 13% having isolated systolic hypertension.

The advantages of treating hypertension in those over 70 are less clear than for younger patients. Some studies have failed to show a correlation between hypertension and excess morbidity and mortality in the elderly. These findings seem odd when compared with the risks shown for younger patients but are difficult to explain away. Secondly, few studies have investigated the benefits of treating raised blood pressure in the very old. Thirdly, the elderly are a population at greater risk from the side effects of drug treatment.

The recent report from the European Working Party on Hypertension in the Elderly (EWPHE) has gone some way towards rectifying these deficiencies.

EWPHE study

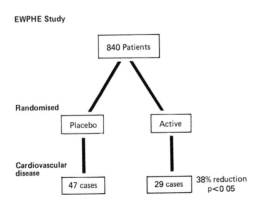

EWPHE Study

840 Patients

Randomised

Placebo

Active

Cardiovascular
disease

47 cases

29 cases

38% reduction
p<0 05

Eight hundred and forty patients aged over 60 (mean 72 years) were included in this multicentre placebo controlled study. The active treatment used (hydrochlorothiazide and triampterene, with methyldopa added if necessary) reflects the fact that the study began in the early 1970's. The study ended in 1984 because of an important reduction (36%) in the number of heart attacks. The incidence of cardiovascular mortality and cerebrovascular disease, but not cerebrovascular mortality, also decreased. These benefits were achieved during this study without a proportional increase in adverse effects from active treatment.

The EWPHE study does not answer all our questions but it does suggest that treating hypertension in the elderly is worth while. When considered together with data from other studies, there is little doubt that patients aged 69 and younger with diastolic pressures of 100 mm Hg and above should be treated. A higher threshold might be acceptable for patients over 70, but treatment is recommended if they meet certain criteria (figure).

Choice of drugs

Contraindications to treatment

Poor general health

Disorders likely to significantly
reduce life expectancy

 Malignancy

 Dementia

Disorders likely to make treatment difficult

 Poor compliance

 Confusion

The choice of drug treatment is based largely on the presence or absence of coexisting disease, which may favour one drug or contraindicate another. As a general rule, treatment should be started with a small dose and gradually increased. The dose regimen should be kept as simple as possible.

Thiazide diuretics are the drugs of choice. They are not without problems, and serum potassium concentrations should be monitored within the first two weeks and thereafter every three to six months. Diabetes mellitus, gout, urinary incontinence, and prostatism are relative contraindications.

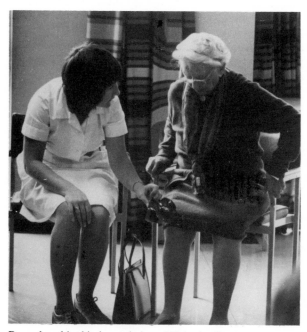

Reproduced by kind permission of Help the Aged

Beta blockers are well tolerated by otherwise fit elderly patients, although the higher prevalence of chest and peripheral vascular disease among the elderly reduces the number of patients to whom they can safely be given. There is some evidence to suggest that they are less effective in older patients but this is not well founded.

Of the calcium antagonists it has been claimed that nifedipine is more effective as an antihypertensive drug in older patients. Verapamil has a greater effect on the heart than nifedipine and should not be used in the presence of heart block or cardiac failure.

There is little information about the use of angiotensin converting enzyme inhibitors in the elderly. Care must be taken with patients already receiving diuretics, but gradually introduced in small doses these drugs seem to be well tolerated.

Methyldopa proved to be both effective and well tolerated in the EWPHE study. There is concern, however, about the central effects (sedation and depression) of this drug, and it is not the drug of first choice for treating the elderly.

HEP study

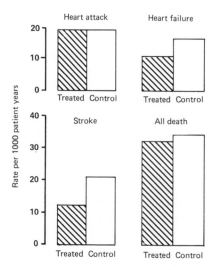

From Beevers DG, MacGregor GA, *Hypertension In Practice*. London: Martin Dunitz, 1987.

In 1986 the results of the primary health care trial of Hypertension in Elderly Patients (HEP) were published.[1] This study confirmed the benefits of antihypertensive treatment in the prevention of stroke, but unlike the findings of the EWPHE study, there was no prevention of heart attacks despite the use of β blockade.

Reference
Coope J, Warrender TS. Randomised trial of treatment of hypertension in elderly patients in primary care. *Br Med J* 1986; 293: 1145–5.

HYPERTENSION IN PREGNANCY

Clinical features of pre—eclamptic toxaemia

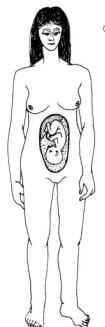

Oedema of face (especially mornings)

High blood pressure at 7th month
(140/100)

Uterus and fetus small for dates

Unreactive cardiotocograph

Rings tight

Proteinuria

Swollen ankles

Blood pressures over 140/100 mm Hg at any stage of pregnancy are associated with a clinically important risk to both mother and baby. In Western countries pre-eclamptic toxaemia is second only to congenital abnormalities as a cause of perinatal death.

About one fifth of all pregnancies are complicated by some form of hypertension. If, in its mildest form, blood pressure stays down there is rarely any increase in risk. Of all hypertensive pregnancies, however, about 2% end with a perinatal death. The risk to the mother is much lower and is more closely related to the presence of underlying renal disease or phaeochromocytoma.

It has never been possible to conduct a large enough clinical trial to prove beyond all doubt that the control of blood pressure in pregnancy is worth while. There is, however, strong evidence from several small studies that indicates the usefulness of antihypertensive treatment in preventing both intrauterine death and intrauterine growth retardation. Both intrauterine growth retardation and intrauterine death are related to placental insufficiency and reduced uterine blood flow.

Syndromes of hypertension in pregnancy

Pre-exsiting essential hypertension

Pre-existing renal disease:
  Pyelonephritis
  Glomerulonrphritis
  Systemic lupus erythematosus

Hypertension induced by pregnancy

Pre-eclamptic toxaemia

Pre-eclamptic toxaemia on
pre-existing hypertension

High risk groups

Teenage mothers
Primigravidae
History of raised blood pressure
Diabetic mothers
Twin pregnancies
Low social class
Rhesus isoimmunisation

Previous oral contraceptive
hypertension (weak association)

The aetiology of pregnancy induced by hypertension and pre-eclampsia is obscure. Abnormalities of the renin angiotensin system, prostaglandins, platelet function, and immunoglobulins have been described, but their clinical importance is uncertain.

There are no reliable markers of placental insufficiency. In severe pre-eclamptic toxaemia proteinuria and oedema occur, and the serum uric acid concentration is raised. Fetal growth can be monitored by several measurements of biparietal diameter and the fetal heart rate in response to spontaneous movements using a cardiotocograph.

Measure blood pressure carefully at first antenatal visit

- Receiving antihypertensive treatment
- Untreated diastolic blood pressure 90 mmHg or more
- Untreated diastolic blood pressure below 90 mmHg

Diastolic blood pressure 100 mmHg or more → Urgent admission for investigation and therapy

Diastolic blood pressure 90–99 mmHg → Outpatient investigation and treatment only

Diastolic blood pressure rises to 90 mmHg or more But no oedema or proteinuria

Serum electrolytes, urine culture, 24 hour urine catecholamines

Adjust treatment to avoid thiazides or ACE inhibitors

Diastolic blood pressure remains over 90 mmHg

Use either atenolol, or labetalol, or methyldopa

Add hydralazine or nifedepine if necessary

Diastolic blood pressure rises to above 90 mmHg, with oedema or proteinuria

Reduce diastolic blood pressure to below 90 mmHg

Aim for full term normal delivery

Diagnose pre-eclampsia

In all but the most severe cases mothers should not be admitted to hospital. Bed rest and tranquilisers have no place in obstetric hypertension. Mothers, who in the antenatal clinic have blood pressures between 130/90 and 140/100 mm Hg, should be rechecked with reliable blood pressure measurement within seven days. Treatment with antihypertensive drugs should be started in the antenatal clinic if the blood pressure exceeds 140/100 mm Hg, or if it is obviously rising.

In obstetric hypertension, unlike all other hypertensive diseases, it is usual to measure diastolic blood pressure at the fourth phase (muffling of sounds). Joint antenatal and hypertension clinics with collaboration between the obstetrician and a physician can lead to efficient and consistent control of blood pressure. Cooperation cards are mandatory to facilitate liaison with district midwives and general practitioners.

No antihypertensive drugs have been reported to be teratogenic. As far as it is known angiotensin converting enzyme inhibitors (captopril and enalapril) should not be used. In late pregnancy diuretic treatment may, by promoting diuresis, cause a further fall in placental blood flow so this group of drugs is usually avoided, unless there is concomitant renal or cardiac failure.

Severe hypertension in pregnancy can kill the mother as well as the baby. Emergency reduction of blood pressure is mandatory if eclampsia is to be avoided: diazepam given intravenously to prevent eclampsia fits and hydralazine intramuscularly (20 mg); or diazoxide given intravenously (50–150 mg); or labetalol infusion (start 20 mg/hour) and emergency delivery by lower segment caesarian section.

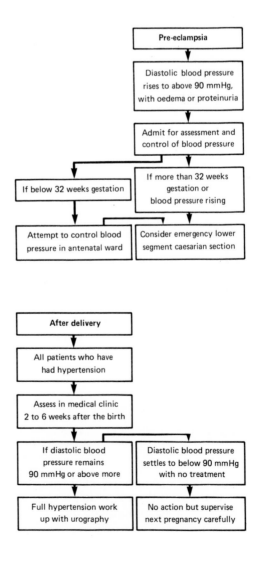

Pre-eclampsia

Diastolic blood pressure rises to above 90 mmHg, with oedema or proteinuria

Admit for assessment and control of blood pressure

- If below 32 weeks gestation → Attempt to control blood pressure in antenatal ward
- If more than 32 weeks gestation or blood pressure rising → Consider emergency lower segment caesarian section

After delivery

All patients who have had hypertension

Assess in medical clinic 2 to 6 weeks after the birth

- If diastolic blood pressure remains 90 mmHg or above more → Full hypertension work up with urography
- Diastolic blood pressure settles to below 90 mmHg with no treatment → No action but supervise next pregnancy carefully

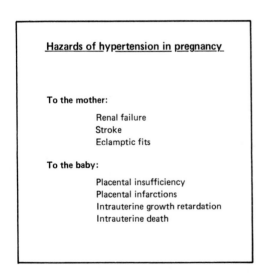

Hazards of hypertension in pregnancy

To the mother:

Renal failure
Stroke
Eclamptic fits

To the baby:

Placental insufficiency
Placental infarctions
Intrauterine growth retardation
Intrauterine death

SUMMARY OF RECENT ADVANCES IN THE TREATMENT OF HYPERTENSION

There is an enormous amount of research into hypertension being carried out in practically every developed country. At present there are no less than five journals exclusively devoted to this topic, and many important papers also appear in the general journals, including the *British Medical Journal*. From a practical point of view the most important advances have been in our understanding of the treatment of mild hypertension and the place of the new classes of antihypertensive drugs in our therapeutic armoury.

The clinical trials

Between 1979 and 1985 several important publications on the treatment of mild hypertension were published. These have been reviewed extensively elsewhere,[1 2] and it is not necessary to restate all the arguments. The Australian National High Blood Pressure Study (ANBPS)[3] and the Hypertension Detection and Follow up Program (HDFP)[4] provided reliable evidence that antihypertensive treatment is effective in preventing strokes in patients with mild hypertension, though the data on coronary prevention were disappointing.

In 1985 the results of three new major treatment trials of mild to moderate hypertension were published. These were the Medical Research Council Mild Hypertension Trial (MRC),[5] the European Working Party Trial of Hypertension in the Elderly (EWPHE),[6] and the International Prospective Primary Prevention Trial of Hypertension (IPPPSH).[7] In 1986 two further trials were conducted, the Heart Attack and Primary Prevention Study (HAPPHY)[8] and the British General Practice Trial of Elderly Patients (HEP).[9]

It had been hoped that many important questions about mild hypertension would have been resolved by the MRC trial, but, in fact, it has posed as many questions as it has answered.

Mild hypertension

It is our view that the MRC trial data, together with those of the ANBPS and the HDFP studies, do provide enough justification for the routine prescription of antihypertensive drugs to patients whose diastolic blood pressures are consistently above 100 mm Hg. The evidence of the benefits of treating patients with diastolic blood pressures between 90 and 99 mm Hg are still insufficient, and here the clinician has to weigh up the possible benefits of treatment against the side effects. Many patients have other problems or conditions that may influence the decision to treat. In particular, the presence of a bad family history must be taken into account.

One issue, highlighted by the MRC trial, is the method of assessing new patients. It is now clear that blood pressures may fall further even after a third pretreatment screening visit. Starting treatment with antihypertensive drugs on the basis of blood pressures measured on only one or two occasions is now totally unacceptable.

There are many other lessons to be learnt from the Medical Research Council trial that will influence the manner of detecting and managing hypertension in general practice, as well as the choice of pharmacological agent. Perhaps the most important message from the trial is that the efficient detection and management of all grades of hypertension can be achieved in the context of the primary health care team. General practice, such as we have in the United Kingdom, is a potentially invaluable source of both epidemiological and pharmacological data: developments in this field must be encouraged.

The elderly

After the publication of the EWPHE and HEP results we now have a clear mandate to prescribe antihypertensive agents in patients up to the age of about 75 years. We still need more information on older patients and we also need to know more of the benefits of treating isolated systolic hypertension. The results of the American Systolic Hypertension in the Elderly Program (SHEP)[10] may be published some time near 1990; preliminary results about the feasibility of reducing systolic pressure are encouraging.

The new data on the elderly have important implications for primary health care as they mean that a great many more people registered with a general practitioner are in need of detection, follow up, and even treatment with drugs. Between one third and one half of all people aged 65 years or more have blood pressures above 160/95 mm Hg at first screening, and although many pressures will settle on rechecking, this must mean an increase in the clinical load on family doctors.

Thiazides

It is also evident from the MRC trial, as well as the EWPHE, ANBPS, and HDFP trials, that the antithiazide propaganda of the past few years has been overstated. Despite the many biochemical side effects and the high incidence of impotence reported by the MRC trial this group of drugs used in low doses is very effective, particularly in older patients. There really is no evidence to suggest that thiazide diuretics increase the risk of coronary heart disease. Another important consideration is that these drugs are cheap.

β blockers

Many people had hoped that the β adrenoceptor blockers would have had advantageous effects over and above that of lowering blood pressure. Beta blockers are known to be effective in the secondary prevention of coronary heart disease, so it was logical to hope that they might have added benefits in primary prevention in patients with hypertension. Both the results of the MRC and IPPPSH trials were at first slightly disappointing, but detailed analysis of subgroups in both studies suggests, but does not prove, that the beneficial effects of metabolised β blockers on coronary prevention may be negated by smoking: "cigarette smoking and β blocker interaction" is of great interest and likely to be the basis of primary research in the future.

Other first line drugs

Since 1980 the development of the calcium entry blockers nifedipine and verapamil[11] and the angiotensin converting enzyme inhibitors captopril and enalapril[12] have widened the choice of first line antihypertensive treatment. These groups of drugs, which are basically vasodilators, seem to be getting nearer to the basic mechanism of hypertension, and their relative lack of side effects means that they may challenge the supremacy of β blockers and thiazides. In many patients, in whom β blockers and thiazides are contraindicated, calcium blockers or angiotensin converting enzyme inhibitors are very attractive alternatives.

Step care

In the first edition of the *ABC of Hypertension* we suggested a fairly simple "step care" method of treating blood pressure. Things are now more complex, so in answer to the question, does it matter how we reduce blood pressure? the answer seems to be no, but the choise of drug depends on potential side effects, and the treatment regimen can be tailored for the individual patient. The basic therapeutic principle remains: we should add second and third line drugs of different classes, rather than using increasing doses of one agent. Step care diagrams are now too complicated to be meaningful and do not take into account the diversity of clinical medicine and the many other possible concomitant diseases.

The role of the nurse

It has become evident from the successful organisation of the MRC trial that nurses, when suitably trained, can detect and manage hypertensive patients very well. In view of the increasing work load, particularly with the treatment of older patients, the efficient use of general practice nurses will be crucial. The British Hypertension Society has chosen to organise regular nurse training sessions, and other organisations have much to contribute in this field. Perhaps the official nurse training schools should also organise tuition, both for students and trained nurses, on the detection and management of hypertension, as well as other chronic diseases.

The bad news

In the early 1970s the "rule of halves" was described. This implied that only a minority of hypertensive people were receiving the treatment they needed. Practically every population study published since has confirmed this woeful picture. Although there is heartening evidence that increasing numbers of general practitioners are making special efforts to detect their hypertensive patients, the national picture has not improved.[13] The only solution to this problem is the indoctrination of young general practitioner trainees in the importance of active screening or case detection programmes in their routine work. Many opinion leaders have advocated this for some years, but still there is evidence of a general poor quality of surveillance and care. While there is no reason to doubt that the primary health care team is still the best place to organise positive health screening, this is not yet universally accepted or organised. Here again the properly trained nurse could have an important part to play.

Summary of recent advances in the treatment of hypertension

Conclusion

Hypertension remains the commonest chronic disease requiring treatment with drugs in the Western world. It can be exciting and rewarding to manage, but the lack of recognition of its importance, both in general practice and in hospitals, is worrying. Good higher medical training is urgently needed.

References
1   Breckenridge A. Treating mild hypertension. *Br Med J* 1985; **291**: 89–90.
2   Moser M, Black H, Stair D. The dilemma of mild hypertension. *Drugs* 1986; **31**: 279–87.
3   Management Committee. The Australian Therapeutic Trial in Mild Hypertension. *Lancet* 1980: i: 1261–7.
4   Hypertension Detection and Follow-up Program Co-operative Group. Five year findings of the hypertension detection and follow-up program: (1) Reduction in mortality of persons with high blood pressure, including mild hypertension. (2) Mortality by race/sex and age. *JAMA* 1979; **292**: 2563–77.
5   Medical Research Council Working Party. MRC trial of mild hypertension, principal results. *Br Med J* 1985; **291**: 97–104.
6   Amery A, Birkenhäger W, Brixko P, *et al*. Mortality and morbidity results from the European Working Party on high blood pressure in the elderly trial. *Lancet* 1985; **i**: 1349–54.
7   The IPPPSH Collaborative Group. Cardiovascular risk and risk factors in a randomised trial of treatment based on the beta-blocker oxprenolol: The International Prospective Primary Prevention Study in Hypertension (IPPPSH). *Journal of Hypertension* 1985; **3**: 379–92.
8   Wilhelmsen L, Berglund G, Elmfeldt O, Wedel A. Beta-blockers versus saluretics in hypertension. Comparison of total mortality, myocardial infarction and sudden death. Study design and early results of blood pressure reduction. *Prev Med* 1981; **10**: 38–45.
9   Coope J, Warrender TS. Randomised trial of treatment of hypertension in elderly patients in primary care. *Br Med J* 1986; **293:** 1145–51.
10 Hully SB, Furbert CD, Gurland B, *et al*. Systolic hypertension in the elderly program (SHEP). Antihypertensive efficacy of chlorthalidone. *Am J Cardiol* 1985; **56**: 913–20.
11 Calcium channel blockers. Proceedings of a symposium. *Am J Med* 1984; 77: symposium issue 2B.
12 ACE converting enzyme inhibitors. Proceedings of a symposium. *Am J Med* 1984; 77: 2A.
13 Coope JR. Hypertension in general practice. What is to be done? *Br Med J* 1984; **288**: 880–1.

DETECTING HYPERTENSIVE PATIENTS

The rule of halves

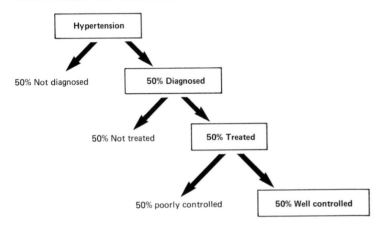

The expression "the rule of halves" aptly expresses the current state of underdiagnosis, undertreatment, and poor control of blood pressure in the general population. This is probably due to a series of dangerous myths about hypertension which are perpetuated despite ample evidence to the contrary.

The myths and the solutions

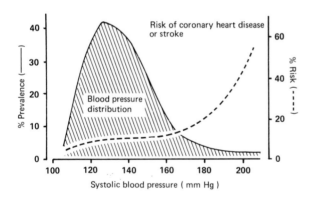

From Wilhelmsen, *Clin Sci*. 1979; **57**: 455–8.

The first myth is that occasional mildly raised blood pressure readings are attributable to minor stresses and can be ignored. The next myth is that hypertensive patients can be relied on to present with diagnostically useful symptoms such as headache and tiredness. An even more dangerous myth is the belief that once drug treatment has adequately reduced blood pressure treatment can be discontinued.

As people with high blood pressure cannot be diagnosed in a casual manner some systematic method of detecting symptomless cases is needed. The only way to do this is to measure blood pressure routinely in all adults, especially those aged over 40. This could be achieved through mass screening exercises, rather like mass radiography in the era of tuberculosis, but this might be expensive and would mean creating new branches of the health services.

Screening

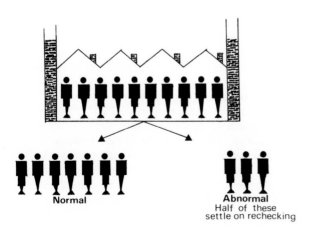

Screening for hypertension at the work place by occupational health doctors has more practical advantages if the relevant information can be transmitted efficiently to those doctors who have the responsibility for prescribing medicines. The current interest in health and safety at work should give added impetus to this approach.

The provision of blood pressure measuring apparatus in shops and supermarkets in the hope of attracting the general population to "have a check" has little to recommend it. It probably attracts only known hypertensive patients, who want a double check, and may induce undue anxiety in people who have a mildly increased risk but in whom treatment with drugs is not justified.

Clinical examination

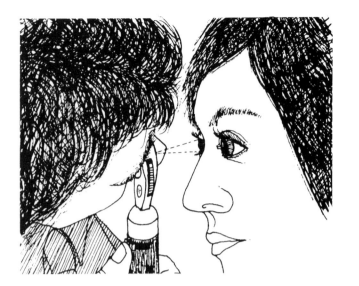

Delayed femoral pulses are present in coarctation of the aorta. Patients with acromegaly or Cushing's syndrome have a distinctive appearance. Polycystic kidneys may be palpable on abdominal examination, and unilateral renal artery stenosis is usually present if a systolic-diastolic bruit is audible lateral to the midline.

There may be clinical evidence of cardiac enlargement or abnormalities of the optic fundi.

Using the ophthalmoscope

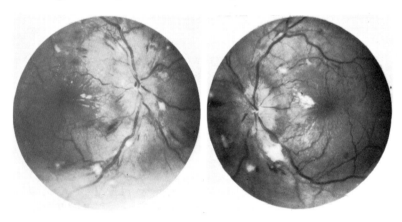

Retinal haemorrhages should be carefully looked for. Bilateral flame shaped haemorrhages indicate malignant hypertension. The appearance of these haemorrhages coincides with the development of fibrinoid necrosis in the arterioles of the kidney.

Cotton wool spots, due to infarction of the nerve fibre layer of the retina, are an ominous sign, as is papilloedema. Hard exudates, which often cluster round the macula, are only slightly less important.

Hyaline degeneration of the arterial wall (indicated by increased light reflex) occurs with aging and with high blood pressure.

X rays and ECGs

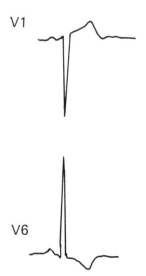

V1

V6

ECG Showing left ventricular hypertrophy

All patients should have a plain radiograph of the chest and an electrocardiogram. Radiology occasionally shows cardiac enlargement and, very rarely, notching on the underside of the ribs caused by collateral vessels in coarctation of the aorta.

The ECG is more sensitive in detecting left ventricular enlargement than x-ray studies. Echocardiography is the best method of detecting ventricular hypertrophy but may not be cost effective. Hypertensive patients who develop evidence of left ventricular hypertrophy on ECG, particularly if accompanied by ST and T wave changes in the leads overlying the left ventricle, are in great jeopardy. The Framingham study showed that 30% of patients with definite left ventricular hypertrophy on ECG die within five years. Patients with such changes should be treated, although high voltage changes alone can sometimes be explained by other factors, such as a thin chest wall in a young subject.

Detecting hypertensive patients

General practice: the secret weapon

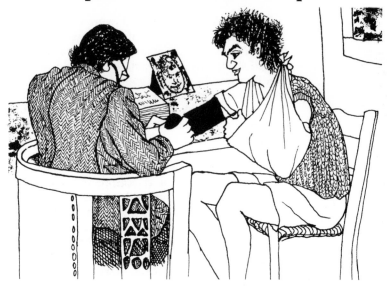

The most obvious solution to the failure of patients to get themselves diagnosed is to use existing health care resources efficiently. In Western countries about 85% of the population see a doctor at least once in three years. Usually patients attend for other reasons, complaining of some specific unassociated symptom. This is the ideal opportunity to measure blood pressure routinely in all comers, no matter what their presenting complaint. It is thus feasible to examine a very large proportion of the adult population without special screening units or equipment.

Who measures the blood pressure?

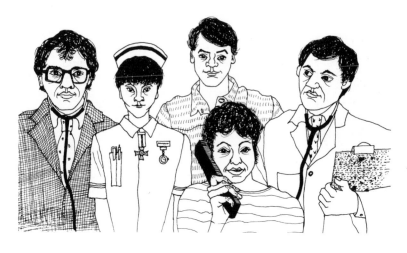

Blood pressure may be measured by the family doctors, the practice nurse, the receptionist, or any suitably trained person. Tuition in measuring blood pressure takes only about half an hour.

Not only family doctors, but all doctors in every branch of medicine—physicians, surgeons, and casualty doctors—have the same responsibility to measure blood pressure in all comers and ensure that any abnormalities are referred to the family doctor.

About 0·5% of the adult population will have very severe hypertension requiring urgent investigation and treatment. This represents no more than five cases for each individual general practitioner. A further 10 to 15% of adults will have pressures above 100 mm Hg and will probably need drug treatment if this level of blood pressure persists. A further 20% of the population will have pressures of 90 to 99 mm Hg, and as they have a measurably increased risk, they will need systematic follow up, even though there is little evidence to show that they need treatment.

Other risk factors

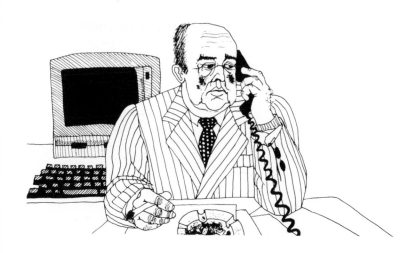

When assessing hypertensive patients, other coronary risk factors should be taken into account. These include obesity, cigarette smoking, physical inactivity, hypercholesterolaemia and alcohol intake. Action to reduce obesity and stop smoking is known to be beneficial. There is no evidence that the treatment of hypercholesterolaemia prolongs life, but the presence of high cholesterol concentrations might lower the threshold above which antihypertensive treatment might be started.

Records

DATE	21/9/85	7/10/85	18/10/85	7/11/85	5/12/85	9/1/86	4 MAR 86	7 MAY 86	4 JULY 86	6/8/86	18/8/86
B.P. Sitting/Lying	184/116	178/114	165/104	158/96	168/98	198/88	142/84.	136/80	148/92	198/100	132/82
PULSE Sitting/Lying	96	92	64	64	60	60	62	62	64	68	76
B.P. Standing	192/122						148/92	140/94	158/100	160/102	138/80
PULSE Standing	100						68	64	64		
WEIGHT kg / st lbs	84 kg	83.5	83.0	83	82	83	82.5 kg	81 Kg	80 Kg	79 kg	79 Kg
DRUG (Dose/Day) 1 ATENOLOL		START 100 mg	100 mg	100 mg	STOP						
DRUG (Dose/Day) 2 (EMOREHC					START TAB I	tab 1	tab ↑	↑	↑	tab I	↑
DRUG (Dose/Day) 3 NIFEDEPINE					↓				start 20mg twice daily	start 20mg twice daily	↑ b.d.
DRUG (Dose/Day) 4											
DRUG (Dose/Day) 5					NURSE FOLLOW-UP CLINIC PLEASE			DR JONES AT NEXT VISIT PLEASE		BACK TO NURSE FOLLOW-UP	
DRUG (Dose/Day) 6											
SERUM UREA	6.7										
SERUM POTASSIUM	4.2										
OTHER INVESTIGATION	Urine Nad						WEIGHT ADVICE				
TIME TO NEXT VISIT	2/52	2/52	3/52	4/52	4/52	2 months	2/12	2/12	1/12	2/52	6/52
DOCTOR's SIGNATURE	GB	K	GB	GB	GB	GB	ANZ	ANZ	ANZ	GB	GB

Efficient detection and follow up of hypertension requires an efficient record system. The existing octavo general practitioner record sheet and folder can, with simple modification, be used to good effect, but A4 records are ideal. Once a general practitioner has decided to embark on a hypertension detection exercise the simplest system is to insert a stiff coloured card into the folder of all adults over 40 years of age. It should remain there until the individual patient has attended and had his blood pressure measured. Record cards for hypertension follow up, with a protruding "flag," are available from many drug companies.

Once the hypertensive patient has been detected a permanent marker, or sticker, or rubber stamp should identify the record folder to remind the doctor of the diagnosis and the need for follow up at each visit.

Screening protocol

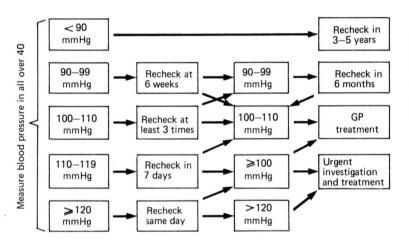

The prime responsibility for the detection and management of hypertension rests in general practice. Efficient reduction in blood pressure definitely prevents both heart attacks and strokes. Thus the time has come to organise the care of hypertension systematically in general practice.

The authors gratefully acknowledge the help of Drs Linda Beeley and Dr Adu.

INVESTIGATION

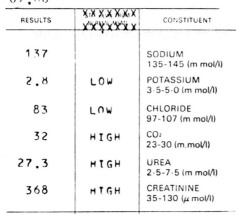

RESULTS	XXXXXXX XXXXXXX	CONSTITUENT
137		SODIUM 135-145 (m mol/l)
2.8	LOW	POTASSIUM 3·5-5·0 (m mol/l)
83	LOW	CHLORIDE 97-107 (m mol/l)
32	HIGH	CO_2 23-30 (m.mol/l)
27.3	HIGH	UREA 2·5-7·5 (m mol/l)
368	HIGH	CREATININE 35-130 (μ mol/l)

Secondary hypertension is rare in patients with raised arterial pressures, and routine screening to detect renovascular and endocrine hypertension shows a poor return. A policy of selection is therefore necessary.

Detailed investigation may be restricted to those patients who:
(a) have malignant hypertension (bilateral retinal haemorrhages),
(b) have poorly controlled blood pressure with adequate doses of the commonly used drugs (not due to non-compliance),
(c) are aged under 30 years,
(d) have an unusual clinical history—for example, sweating attacks,
(e) have abnormal plasma concentrations of urea, creatinine, or potassium,
(f) have positive urine tests for protein, blood, or sugar,
(g) have a rapid rise in blood pressure or an abdominal bruit.

Investigations for all patients

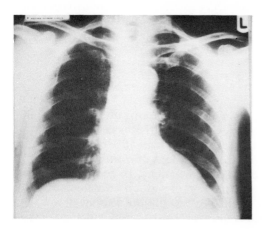

Does the average middle aged patient with mild to moderately raised arterial pressure need any tests? Some patients in Britain are treated by their family doctors without initial biochemical or radiological investigations, but a limited number of tests are justified. These should include an examination of the optic fundi, an electrocardiogram, a plain chest radiograph, and simple blood and urine tests.

Tests are also useful for identifying other risk factors for vascular disease. It is also important to look for evidence of damage to "target" organs, though treatment must not be left until such damage occurs. Many patients with high blood pressure have no symptoms or signs until a cardiovascular catastrophe occurs.

History

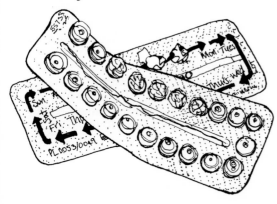

It is important to ask about a family history of stroke or primary hypertension.

In phaeochromocytoma there may be attacks of sweating, throbbing headache, or palpitations; in primary aldosteronism muscle weakness, polyuria, or paraesthesia; and in Cushing's syndrome rapid weight gain or spontaneous bruising.

What about oral contraceptives?
In most women the oestrogen containing pill causes a small rise in arterial pressure and in some the rise may be pronounced; in rare instances malignant hypertension may develop. The effect is smaller but still present with the lower dose preparations. The progestagen minipill, a less effective contraceptive, has little effect on blood pressure.

Urine tests

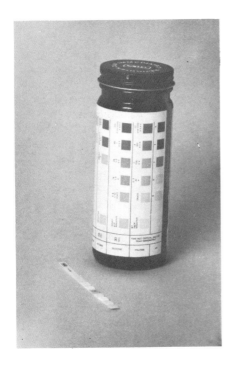

Tests using reagent strips ("Stix" tests) of urine for blood, protein, and sugar are easy to perform but all too often omitted. The test for blood becomes more sensitive if red cells in urine are lysed with a drop of detergent.

Proteinuria or haematuria in the absence of malignant hypertension suggests underlying renal disease, such as glomerulonephritis. Urine microscopy is necessary in patients with positive strip test results, but the value of routine urine culture in the absence of either a positive strip test result or a history suggesting urinary tract infection is doubtful: it is unlikely to be of value in men.

If a patient has blood pressures that fluctuate widely, increase with drug treatment, or show a pronounced postural fall then urinary catecholamine metabolites or plasma noradrenaline concentrations should be measured.

Maturity onset diabetes and raised arterial pressure are common conditions that often coexist in patients who are overweight. Blood pressure must be carefully controlled in diabetics as high pressure accelerates the development of retinopathy. Only rarely are diabetes and high blood pressure caused by endocrine diseases such as phaeochromocytoma, Cushing's syndrome, and acromegaly. Mild impairment of glucose tolerance is common in patients with primary aldosteronism but is corrected by treatment. Thiazide diuretics may precipitate or worsen diabetes mellitus.

Blood tests

16.00

RESULTS	STD DEV'N FROM NORMAL MEAN	CONSTITUENT
145	HIGH	SODIUM 136-144 (m mol/l)
2.6	LOW	POTASSIUM 3.4-4.9 (m mol/l)
105		CHLORIDE 95-105 (m mol/l)
29	HIGH	CO_2 21-28 (m mol/l)
3.8		UREA 2.5-7.0 (m mol/l)
71		CREATININE 35-115 (μ mol/l)

Measurement of serum potassium concentrations is a simple screening test for patients with primary aldosteronism, although false negative results may occur.

Plasma renin activity is usually very low in primary aldosteronism, but up to 30% of patients with essential hypertension also have subnormal values. Patients with low renin primary hypertension respond well to thiazide diuretics.

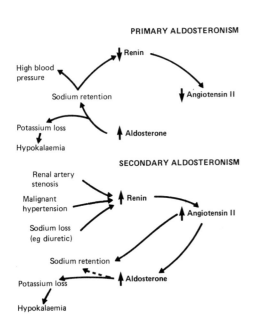

PRIMARY ALDOSTERONISM

SECONDARY ALDOSTERONISM

In primary aldosteronism (or in other rare forms of mineralocorticoid hypertension such as 11-β-hydroxylation deficiency and liquorice ingestion) the typical electrolyte picture includes hypokalaemia, increased serum concentrations of bicarbonate, and slightly increased plasma sodium concentrations. In contrast, patients with aldosterone excess due to depletion of sodium or malignant hypertension often have low normal or low plasma sodium concentrations with increased concentrations of renin and angiotensin II.

Thiazide diuretics cause a fall in the serum concentration of potassium that is related to dose: severe hypokalaemia with muscle paralysis may result from the administration of diuretics to patients with primary aldosteronism. Serum or plasma potassium concentrations should be measured before the start of drug treatment on venous samples taken without exercise of the forearm.

Raised plasma concentrations of urea and creatinine occur in patients with impaired renal function owing either to primary renal disease or to renal damage from severe hypertension. Retention of sodium is often a factor in the pathogenesis of the high blood pressure that accompanies renal impairment; thiazide diuretics are relatively ineffective in this condition, and loop diuretics, such as frusemide administered twice a day, are usually necessary.

Investigation

Renovascular hypertension

Right renal artery stenosis
Small kidney size
Delayed dye appearance
Increased contrast density in the collecting system
Delayed washout of contrast after diuresis

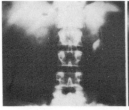 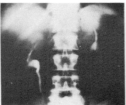 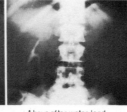

| 2 minutes | 10 minutes | 1 hour after water load |

This simple scheme of investigation will fail to detect the cause in most patients with renovascular hypertension. Narrowing of a renal artery usually results from atheroma in older patients and from fibromuscular hyperplasia in young women. An intravenous urogram (or digital subtraction angiogram when available) is usually necessary, but the routine use of this test in all patients with hypertension is expensive and unrewarding. It is worth investigating only those patients who (a) have poorly controlled blood pressure with drug treatment; (b) have bilateral retinal haemorrhages; or (c) have a rapid rise in blood pressure or an abdominal bruit (d) have impaired renal function; (e) are under 25 years; (f) have widespread atherosclerosis.

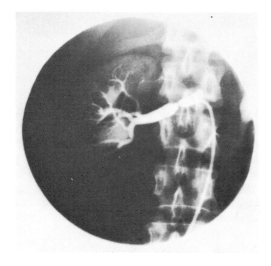

Other screening procedures such as isotope renography or measurements of plasma renin activity may be used. Modern isotopic renography is sensitive but may give false positive results. With renin, false positive and false negative results may occur.

Intravenous urography may show a non-functioning kidney, which can result from occlusion of the renal artery. Such changes may wrongly be attributed to pyelonephritis or hypoplasia unless angiography is carried out.

Since up to 10% of the middle aged population of this country have raised blood pressures investigations should be kept to a minimum in most patients.

MANAGEMENT OF HYPERTENSION IN GENERAL PRACTICE

It is important to remember that hypertension is only one of the known risk factors for cardiovascular disease. To be able to identify those patients at high risk and take appropriate action a general practitioner ideally needs the following information to be present in the records of all patients (especially men) between the ages of 30 and 80:

(*a*) family history of cardiovascular disease,
(*b*) a blood pressure recording within the last five years,
(*c*) current smoking status,
(*d*) weight for height.

In addition, a random serum cholesterol value is desirable, especially for those with other risk factors.

In most practices that have not screened their patients such information will not be held in at least half of the patients. A systematic attempt to bridge this gap should be made.

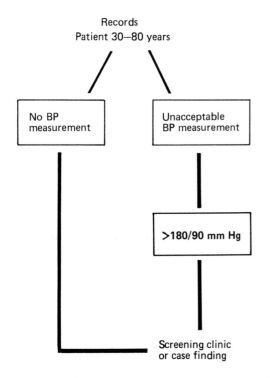

Family history

Blood pressure

Smoking

Weight

Methods of screening

Screening the records—To define the problem the records need to be screened. This may be done by an instructed filing clerk or retired nurse. An age-sex register will cut down the work but is not absolutely necessary. The aim is to find records without acceptable levels of blood pressure recorded during the previous five years. "Acceptable" means below 180 mm Hg systolic and 90 mm Hg diastolic (phase 5) below the age of 65 and below 180/100 mm Hg (phase 5) above this age. The record envelopes can be generally tidied up and pruned at the same time.

Screening the patients—Several methods of measuring the blood pressure of those in need are available, including screening clinics and case finding. For screening clinics patients are sent cards to attend the medical centre at a particular time. This takes dedication but is rewarding and is popular with patients; about three quarters turn up. The practice nurse can inquire about family history, survey smoking habits, measure the blood pressure, measure weight and height, test the urine for glucose, and take a blood sample for serum cholesterol estimation.

The case finding method uses attendances of patients for other reasons. When they are screened the records of those patients who need their blood pressure measured must be marked. If the doctor or nurse is to measure the blood pressure at the same time as the patient attends for something else the most effective reminder is to write "Take BP/smoking/weight/family history" on the next line of the continuation card. A stamp or printed sticker may be used. If the reception staff have to offer a separate appointment for blood pressure examination then a slat should be inserted into the record or a sticker attached to the front. (The slats may be made from laminated plastic $8\frac{1}{2}$ inches × $1\frac{1}{2}$ inches.) Notices or posters advising patients to have their blood pressure measured may be put in the waiting room.

Patients found to have blood pressures above treatment levels (see below) should be told that their pressure is on the high side but that they will need more readings to decide whether they need treatment. They are asked to book five more attendances with the practice nurse and then to make an appointment to see the doctor for evaluation.

Records
Patient 30–80 years

No BP measurement

Unacceptable BP measurement

>180/90 mm Hg

Screening clinic or case finding

Management of hypertension in general practice

Action

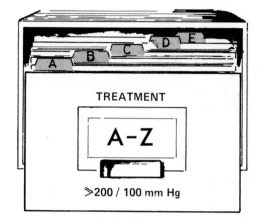

The fact that blood pressure is recorded does not necessarily mean that appropriate action is taken. A search of the records will disclose known hypertensive patients not having treatment, and some patients who do not need treatment will need periodic review. To simplify decision making a "three box" system is useful.

The first box contains those patients who need treatment. It includes:

All those up to the age of 80 with a mean blood pressure from five consecutive attendances of at least 200 mm Hg systolic or 100 mm Hg diastolic (phase 5).

These patients need investigating, as indicated in previous chapters in this book, and should be treated. Thereafter they should be reviewed not less than every six months. A card index file of these patients is maintained and checked against the record cards every six months to make sure the patient is still attending.

The second box contains the patients who need surveillance and includes all those below the age of 80 with blood pressures below those of patients in the first box but above 180/90 mm Hg on any one occasion. A separate card index file is maintained on these patients and they are asked to return for review of their blood pressure every year.

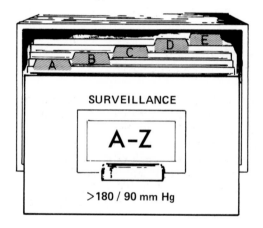

The third box contains patients with blood pressures below those in the second box. No card index file is kept and no regular effort is needed to review these patients. They should have repeat examinations every five years until 80, when their surveillance may be discontinued.

Once the initial screening has examined and classified patients in terms of blood pressure the same method may be used to screen new entrants to the practice and patients who have reached their 35th birthday. The level of blood pressure ascertainment will thus be kept high over the years.

Such a programme might seem ambitious but may be achieved quite easily with the use of a trained nurse to take much of the load from the doctor. The effectiveness of surveillance and treatment may also be monitored periodically.

The hypertension clinic

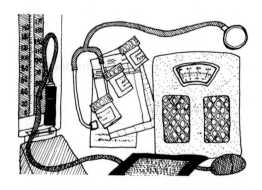

Most practices have an antenatal clinic where patients' progress is reviewed systematically and where much of the work is done by nurses. The same can apply to a hypertension clinic. Blood pressure estimations, weighing, and other tests (such as urine tests) may be done by the nurse before the doctor sees the patient. This leaves the doctor free to review the effectiveness of treatment and discuss side effects or other risk factors such as smoking, alcohol intake, obesity and hypercholesterolaemia.

Reducing blood pressure without attending to these factors is unlikely to be effective in reducing the incidence of heart attacks and stroke. The importance of stopping smoking is paramount. All hypertensive patients should be instructed in the reduction of saturated fat in their diet. Patients who need help in modifying their diet or stopping smoking should be followed up more intensively by the nurse, at first on a weekly basis.

HYPERTENSION

SURNAME	FORENAMES	DATE OF BIRTH
SMITH	Herbert	14·11·28

ADDRESS *the Smithy, Cow Lane.*

SUMMARY OF HISTORY

1978. Discovered during case finding. No family history.

SMOKING HISTORY *Pipe smoker   2oz/week*

ANTIDEPRESSIVE *nil*	STEROIDS *nil*	CONTRACEPTIVE —

BASIC DATA   DATE *20·5·78*

B.P. *180/115*	F.B.C. *normal*	CHOLESTEROL *5·6*
WEIGHT *15 sT.*	Na *134*	LIPOPROTEIN —
FUNDI ✓ ✓	K *39*	LAB URINE ✓
HEART FAILURE ✓	UREA *4·5*	E.C.G. ✓
ABDOMINAL BRUIT *nil*	CREATININE *88*	CHEST FILM ✓
FEMORAL PULSES ✓ ✓	BL. SUGAR —	I.V.P. ✓

ANNUAL REVIEW	79	80
FUNDI	✓	✓
HEART FAILURE	✓	✓
UREA	—	—
CHEST FILM	—	—

Patients who fail to turn up at the clinic are more important than those who appear. They should be sent a reminder or, in exceptional circumstances, be visited by the nurse. In any event the non-attendance should be noted in the record. Failure to continue with treatment ise a common and serious problem.

A card for recording basic data on hypertensive patients and for graphical representation of blood pressure is useful. This enables the doctor to see at a glance what tests have been done and whether the patient's blood pressure is responding to treatment.

Compliance and education

Communication between doctor and patient is very important. Full information should be given to patients before they start treatment in words they can understand. An information sheet is a useful aid. Such sheets can be obtained from some pharmaceutical companies but one produced by the doctor himself is more effective. The points to be included are: the lack of symptoms with hypertension; the reasons for treatment; the need for continuous treatment; the importance of stopping smoking, controlling weight, and reducing salt intake; and the necessity of regular review. Complete openness about blood pressure readings is desirable. The doctor should discuss his success or failure in achieving the blood pressure goals. This fosters a sense of trust that will lead to good compliance. A take it or leave it attitude will often result in the patient opting for the latter. Good working relationships will take months or even years to develop but such a perspective is natural to general practice. The doctor must develop a sensitivity to the patient's symptoms, even when they are not thought to be due to treatment, and there must be readiness to compromise and bargain rather than break off relationships. The use of a practice nurse may also encourage the development of an effective rapport. Patients may confide problems to her that they would not disclose to the doctor. Above all, fear must not be inculcated or the patient allowed to adopt an invalid role, so replacing one disease with another more serious.

SOME NOTES ON BLOOD PRESSURE

Everybody has blood pressure. Without it blood would not flow round the body. When we exercise it goes up when we are sleeping it is very low. During ordinary activities it goes up and down all the time and is regulated by complicated bits of apparatus designed to keep blood flowing to areas of the body that need it. If the blood pressure gets too low the first organ to suffer is the brai...
out. A...

---

3. Do not add salt to your food at table as it encourages blood pressure to rise

Lead a normal life. Take a reasonable amount of exercise. The rise in blood pressure that occurs during exercise involving movement (running, swimming and walking) is not dangerous. Static exercises like weight lifting and press-ups however are not so safe. Do not worry about your blood pressure. Our aim in the blood pressure clinic is to keep all the patients happy until their eightieth birthday. After that we are not making any promises!